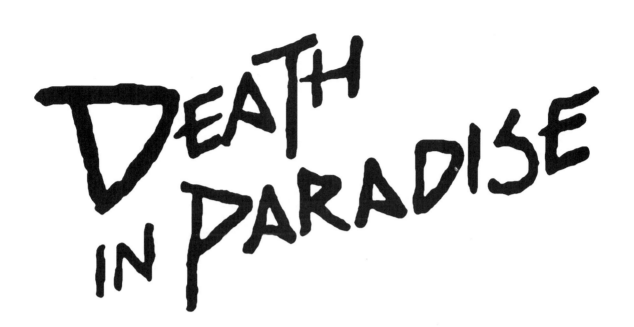

Death in Paradise

An Illustrated History
of the Los Angeles County
Department of Coroner

By Tony Blanche and Brad Schreiber

General Publishing Group
Los Angeles

The original sign for HOLLYWOODLAND was erected in 1923 as a real estate promotion. Peg Entwhistle came down, to her death, from the 50-foot H in 1932; the LAND came down in 1949. To the north, the San Fernando Valley begins to blossom.

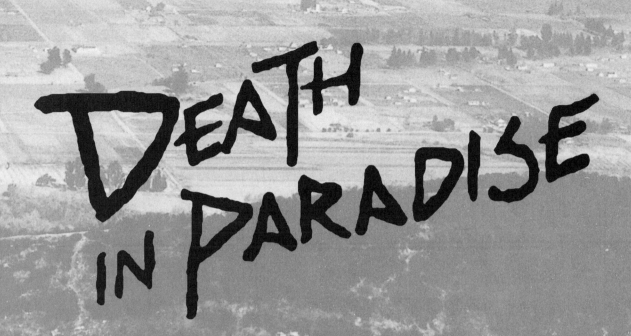

Death in Paradise

An Illustrated History of the Los Angeles County Department of Coroner

By Tony Blanche and Brad Schreiber

Foreword by Anthony T. Hernandez

GPG
GENERAL
PUBLISHING
GROUP, INC

General Publishing Group
Los Angeles

Publisher: W. Quay Hays

Editorial Director: Peter L. Hoffman

Editor: Steve Baeck

Designer: Dana Granoski

Cover Design: Kurt Wahlner

Production Director: Trudihope Schlomowitz

Color and Prepress Manager: Bill Castillo

Production Artist: Bill Neary

Production Assistants: Tom Archibeque, Dave Chadderdon, Russel Lockwood

Editorial Assistant: Dominic Friesen

For information:

General Publishing Group, Inc.
2701 Ocean Park Blvd., Suite 140
Santa Monica, CA 90405

Library of Congress Cataloging-in-Publication Data

Blanche, Tony.
  Death in paradise : an illustrated history of the Los Angeles County Department of Coroner / by Tony Blanche and Brad Schreiber.
     p.   cm.
  ISBN 1-57544-075-X (hc)
  1. Los Angeles County (Calif.). Dept. of Chief Medical Examiner -Coroner--History. 2. Forensic pathology--California--Los Angeles County. I. Schreiber, Brad. II. Title.
RA1063.4.B56   1998
614'.1--dc21   98-21620
                                                                  CIP

Printed in the USA by RR Donnelley & Sons Company

10 9 8 7 6 5 4 3 2 1

General Publishing Group

Los Angeles

Table of Contents

ACKNOWLEDGMENTS

This book owes its existence to Marilyn Lewis, the now-retired marketing coordinator for Skeletons in the Closet at the Los Angeles County Department of Coroner. Her warm response to our first inquiry regarding an illustrated history of the Coroner's Office began it all.

Soon, many of her colleagues were lending support and guidance: Anthony Hernandez, the director at the Department of Coroner who blessed the project throughout; Craig Harvey, chief of operations; Scott Carrier, public information officer; Gary Siglar, retired supervising criminalist; Janie Ito, chief of public services; James Njavro, head of forensic photo and support; Mark Johnson, autopsy supervisor; Joe Muto, chief of the laboratory division; Steve Dowell, research criminalist; David Whiteman, medical examiner; and Esther Benquechea, who cheerfully responded to all our frequent telephone calls.

Dr. Thomas Noguchi, the department's chief medical examiner-coroner from 1967 to 1982, provided special insights and stories, all with good humor, as did the present-day chief medical examiner-coroner, Dr. Lakshmanan Sathyavagiswaran.

Outside the Coroner's Office came invaluable advice regarding photographic and historical sources from Hynda Rudd at the Los Angeles City Archives. Her counsel led us to others to whom we are much indebted: Carolyn Cole, Los Angeles Public Library; Dacey Taub, University of Southern California, Regional History Center; Jean Bruce Poole and William Estrada, El Pueblo de Los Angeles Historical Monument; Katharine Donahue, UCLA's Louise M. Darling Biomedical Library; Alan Jutzi, The Huntington Library; and Marc Wanamaker, Bison Archives.

Beyond these initial sources we discovered two sources, both of whom preserve the best of L.A.'s Chandleresque traditions: photographer Delmar Watson, and investigative reporter and photographer Don Ray.

Anthony Mostrom provided key editorial materials on several cases, particularly the once-infamous 1927 Parker–Hickman case.

Brad Schreiber and I thank Sandra Watt (who provided the glue to keep this book together through uncertain waters) and our always supportive editor, Steve Baeck.

The most appreciation, however, is reserved for our first researcher and collaborator, Tom Burkett, who worked closely with me throughout the first stages of the book. His talents in seeking out a good story and in listening to my old-fashioned ideas about Los Angeles inform the entire project.

—Tony Blanche

With love to my father, Andrew, my sisters, Julie and Robin, my nephews, Justin and Mike, and my common-law stepmom, Donna.

Also, to those whose continued support has been crucial to my career, spirit, and growth as creative artist: Karen Greyson, Peter Hay, Karen Kondazian, Roy Morris, Jim McMullan, J. T. O'Hara, Carol Page, Bill Ratner, Tristine Rainer, Carrie Snow, Nathan Stein, Mike Tunison, Chris Vogler, and, especially, Rick Rees.

—Brad Schreiber

PHOTO SOURCES

Los Angeles County Department of Coroner
pages 16, 19, 20, 33, 34, 42, 43, 63–65, 97, 125
left, 140, 141, 148–151, 158, 163, 165–166, 185

AP/Wide World Photos
pages 116, 117, 127, 146, 152–154

California Historical Society
Title Insurance and Trust Photo Collection
Department of Special Collections
University of Southern California Library
pages 53, 54, 59 bottom, 60

Henry Diltz
page 139

El Pueblo de Los Angeles Historical
Monument
pages 47, 48, 50, 51, 52, 55

Hearst Newspaper Collection
Special Collections
University of Southern California Library
pages 99, 100

Herald Examiner Collection
Los Angeles Public Library
pages 83, 85, 107, 109, 112, 119, 128, 130 bottom,
131, 132

Los Angeles Public Library
pages 86 (Underwood and Underwood), 129
(AP), 130 top (UPI Telephoto)

Don Ray Photo
page 37 bottom

Security Pacific National Bank Photograph
Collection/Los Angeles Public Library
pages 38, 39

Gerald Vale, D.D.S.
pages 167, 168

Marc Wanamaker / Bison Archives
pages 2–3, 89, 120, back jacket (Hollywoodland
sign)

Delmar Watson Photography-Archives, Inc.
pages 12, 15, 36, 37 top, 59 top, 61, 67, 68, 70–73,
74–76, 79–81, 91–93, 95, 96, 98, 103, 104–106,
108, 123, 124, 125 right, 126, 134, 142–144, 159,
179, 180, 181, 182

FOREWORD

For many years, the Los Angeles County Department of Coroner has faced the daunting task of determining the cause and manner of death for those who fall under its jurisdiction. As this book will detail, many cases become scientific odysseys that challenge each individual intimately involved in a given matter and push them to the furthest reaches of their skills and abilities.

It is, after all, to every individual that has ever worked the "front lines" or the "ditches" of death investigation to whom we all owe so much. The Coroner's Office is here to serve the living by providing answers about death, even when the answers are not apparent. It is rare that you would find a Coroner employee at the receiving end of a hero's recognition even though their work is heroic.

Death in Paradise is a humble attempt at shedding light on not only the heroic individuals who have dedicated themselves to finding the truth about death, but also a look at what goes on in the intimate settings of determining why and how someone died. While this book is designed to entertain, it will certainly educate you about the realities of death and its emotional as well as legal significance.

Needless to say, there were countless fascinating and intriguing case histories from which to choose, going as far back as the 19th century when Los Angeles was called El Pueblo de la Reina de Los Angeles. The selected cases were not only highly visible in their time but contain an alluring forensic story that captivates the imagination with the science of death investigation.

We hope that you will find this book to be a rich historical perspective as well as a testament to the Department of Coroner's ongoing commitment to always serve the Los Angeles County community with dignity, respect, and compassion.

— Anthony T. Hernandez
Director, Department of Coroner

PROLOGUE

How They Die

The blood-dimmed tide is loosed, and everywhere
the ceremony of innocence is drowned:
The best lack all conviction, while the worst
are full of passionate intensity.

        —William Butler Yeats, *The Second Coming*

From afar, Los Angeles seems to glow with the exotic aura of the world's most famous fallen cities. It shimmers with the sun-kissed mysteries of Athens, glitters with the riches of Alexandria, and steams with the decadence of Babylon. It's the city of fulfillment, a palm-lined Mediterranean dream gleaming out toward a baby blue sea, where, supposedly, wealth is found daily, fame is bestowed nightly, and identities are reinvented upon arrival.

But for some in Los Angeles, dreams blur with nightmares. Hastily gained prosperity spirals into perversity, instant celebrity fades into delusion, and thoughtless reinvention spawns degeneration. Over the years, this sunbaked, smog-choked paradise has watched, sometimes indifferently, as moguls murder their mistresses, movie stars slash their wrists, and musicians inject fatal overdoses.

Every day, the coroner sweeps up the tragic consequences of this otherworldly madness and sees firsthand what the real-world Los Angeles world denies. In L.A., the city of dreams, the utopia of its imagination cannot overcome its own often-grim reality.

What then is the collective consequence of all this havoc? The daily tally speaks with harsh clarity: Around 200 people die in Los Angeles County each day. Some go peacefully, surrounded by family and friends. They have quiet funerals in suburban chapels, and polished hearses carry them to tranquil cemeteries where their eternal rest is as calm as the breezes that caress their headstones.

For some, however, their spirits continue to haunt their former utopia: the woman and her friend found slashed to death outside her Brentwood townhouse; the sitcom star who shoots himself in his Westwood condo; the pregnant actress knifed to death in a ritual murder at her Bel Air estate; the presidential candidate assassinated at the Ambassador Hotel; the struggling starlet discovered severed at the waist in a weedy lot at the corner of 39th and Norton. These deaths and others like them have left an indelible legacy in the consciousness of Angelenos, leaving them to ponder whether they live in a blessed Eden or its cursed flip side.

Here is L.A., wedged against the Pacific at the bottom corner of the nation, with no choice but to aspire to be more than its surroundings would allow. It started as a sunny desert outpost with a limited freshwater supply. And to make that leap from small city to metropolitan icon, it swindled land from farmers, swiped water rights from neighboring counties, and constructed an elaborate aqueduct to channel it. It drained the Owens

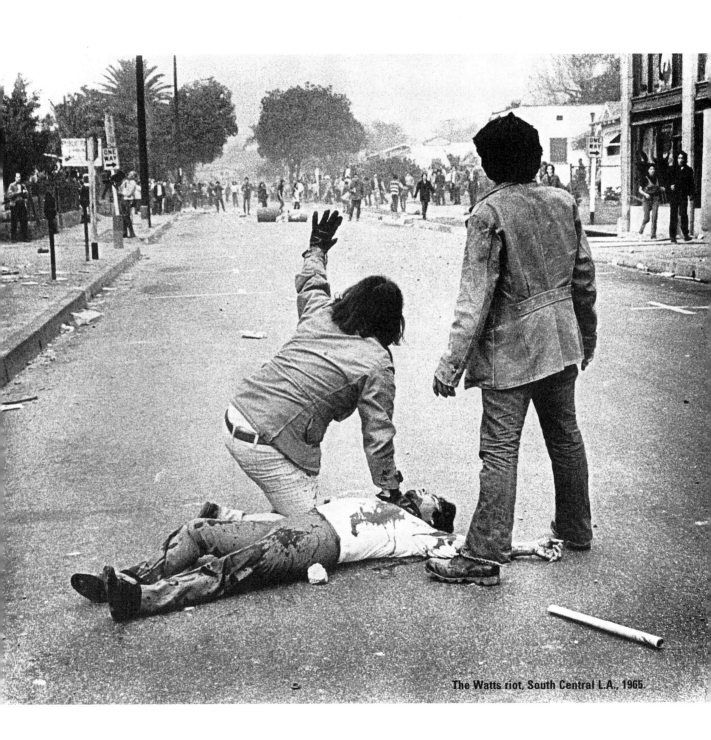

The Watts riot, South Central L.A., 1965.

Valley dry; diverted the Colorado River; and paved over riverbeds, flood plains, and fault lines. Its laconic-paced, easy-living image belies the brutal power, politics, greed, and self-delusion that built it.

This metropolis of over nine million souls now ranks as an international megalopolis brimming with glamour, wealth, and action. But during its climb to the top, in its quest to become a shimmering ideal of the millennium, something in its already faulted foundation was knocked further off-kilter. At its traffic-snarled urban core, commuters in eight-cylinder, high-performance driving machines crawl along in second gear; gleaming corporate towers shadow garment-industry sweatshops; exclusive, gated communities are patrolled by $5-an-hour guards who live in neighboring ghettos that have exploded with rebellion twice in the past 30 years.

In its suburban ring, which sprawls into the foothills, displaced coyotes prowl for small dogs and unattended infants. Autumn fires spread from the brush to the cookie-cutter housing tracts. Winter rains follow, sending two-story homes sliding down muddy slopes. All the while, the distant Owens Valley is dying a dusty death. Deep in the desert, the Colorado River is running dry. The aqueducts are cracking and fault lines are straining and shifting.

But people continue to flock to L.A., despite its ills. Southern California seems to represent the final way station in the quest for the American dream. The promise of Hollywood celebrity, a quick buck, and the redefinition of self is a lure that never seems to fade. It's here where people hope that, someday, busloads of Midwesterners will ogle their mansions; that the offspring of Japanese industrialists will finger their footprints outside the former Grauman's Chinese Theater; that European teenagers will lay roses at their graves.

Of the throngs drawn to the city's charms, a few do in fact achieve fortune, fame, and reinvention. But often, those same few find their dreams remain incomplete, that riches and acclaim have failed to provide the intangible thing they seek.

That's why unnatural celebrity deaths and unnaturally celebrated murders seem to pockmark L.A.'s history with the same randomness that strip malls mar its landscape.

Beyond the daily, sensational television and newspaper reports of the latest tragedy, there is the grim reality of Coroner's Office files. What the world and Angelenos see and hear is sandwiched and blended between weather and traffic updates, sports, news, and political posturing. Gleaming news anchors and stately journalists parade these tragedies as if a yearlong Rose Parade. One is hard-pressed after a while to sort out entertainment from reality: news, documentary simulations, advertising, prime-time silliness, and tragedy all come together into one band of light.

When one reverses this light, back through the prism of the mind, it doesn't refract and form a distinct spectrum. The colors have been lost and we simply move on, feeding at each new turn on more sensation.

However, what one finds at the simple off-white buildings of the coroner's offices in East Los Angeles brings the grim realities back, and into focus. After days of leafing through the yellowed, tattered pages of case files—investigators' reports, police and

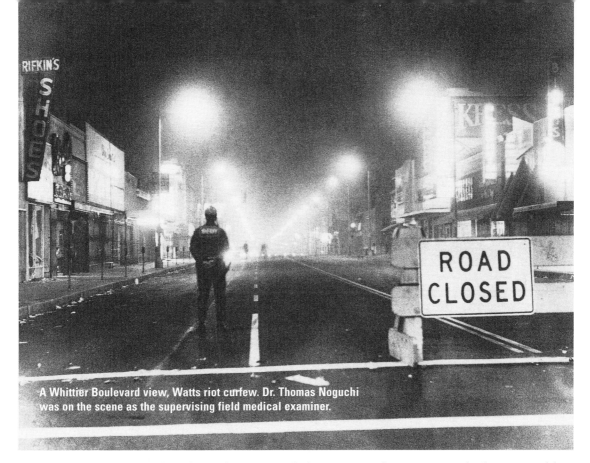

A Whittier Boulevard view, Watts riot curfew. Dr. Thomas Noguchi was on the scene as the supervising field medical examiner.

medical forms, transcripts from the coroner's inquests and autopsy analysis—something else happens. The sadness, the fragility, and irrationality of the events take on medical explanation, psychological motivation.

Reading these files brings one face to face with cold facts that may provide insight where journalistic flamboyance may have failed.

And who presides over this macabre scene? Surprisingly, refreshingly, it is a very matter-of-fact, reasonably cheery group. They include medical, investigative, scientific, and administrative professionals who are keenly aware of their responsibilities to fact-finding, complex procedures, and protecting the privacy of victims' families and friends.

There is light humor in some quarters, but always with two caveats: respect for the

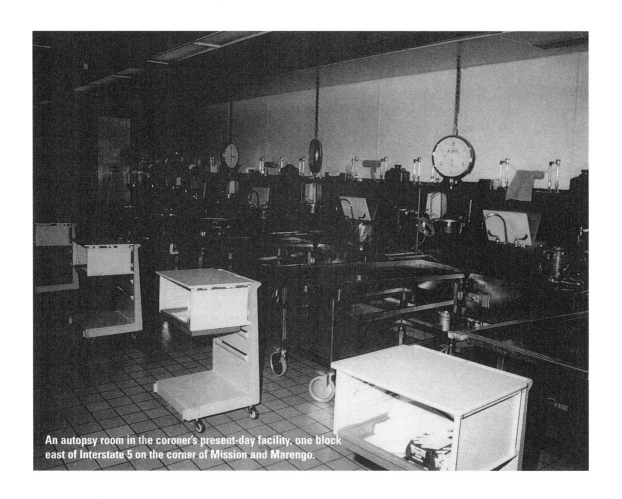

An autopsy room in the coroner's present-day facility, one block east of Interstate 5 on the corner of Mission and Marengo.

deceased and their dearest, and the admission that if a little humor wasn't exchanged, they would all go bonkers. So, within this lugubrious setting, one also comes in contact with a gentle, life-affirming humanism from people uncelebrated, who daily perform routine yet difficult tasks.

What are these tasks? Many are the predictable, necessary bureaucratic and clinical ones. Others, more specific to the institution, call for a unique brand of photography, incisions, weighing of organs and parts, and on-site investigations.

There are highly specialized procedures, such as jaw removal in order to fully analyze dental records, or finger rehydration in order to recapture a full set of fingerprints.

The photography is alarmingly straightforward, nothing purposely sensational, just simple documentation of the body, wounds, and selected body parts or organs, if important to the autopsy record. The photos of Lana Turner's boyfriend, mobster Johnny Stompanato, reveal a body that could be of any slightly built, olive-skinned victim. He is seen unclothed from the waist up with a knife wound in his torso. One is struck by his unmuscular shoulders and arms, a frailty in death which suggests that behind all the bravado of his public persona was a relatively weak man.

Early each morning, the photography staff, 20 or more doctors, and accompanying technicians begin their work of some 20-plus autopsies each day. The popular movie image of bodies in drawers is misleading. They are to be found instead in several large, cold storage rooms where they will stay on average up to three days. Homicides and extraordinarily newsworthy cases are often given priority.

For nonhomicide cases, there is a routine protocol which has four levels of complexity, depending on the circumstances of the death. The first is a complete autopsy, with full toxicology, as if a homicide case. These are mostly celebrated cases of unusual, unwitnessed deaths which are not judged homicides.

The second level is for accidental deaths, e.g., unwitnessed traffic or other accidents.

For these, blood and urine tests seek the presence of alcohol or drugs, but not all toxicology analyses are necessary.

The third is a limited autopsy with limited toxicology. This is for witnessed deaths or suicides accompanied by a note and without complicating factors. For these, stomach contents and blood and/or urine tests are done to confirm the witness reports or suicide note.

The fourth level is an external examination only, with blood and urine toxicology. These are for natural deaths in known circumstances, without a doctor in attendance.

The full homicide protocol is lengthy and complex, beginning with photography. If the case involves gunshot wounds, then fluoroscopy or x-raying is used to determine if there are any foreign objects within. Next, the doctor and technician begin an external examination with a diagram of any scars, marks, tattoos, and injuries.

When this is complete, the internal examination begins, often with a police detective or investigator present. This begins with a Y incision in the chest and the opening of the rib cage. The internal organs are removed one by one so they can be measured, weighed, and analyzed.

This is followed by removal of the neck organs, including the tongue and main arteries. Once this is done, the skull is opened with a lateral ear-to-ear incision so as to remove the skull cap. The brain is weighed and examined for trauma and any abnormalities.

By now, the doctor and technician have collected and preserved any tissues to be saved for later investigation and judicial procedures. The protocol is now complete; the parts are put back, and the body is stitched, washed, wrapped, and sent off to a mortuary where it can regain some semblance of dignity, ready for final commemoration.

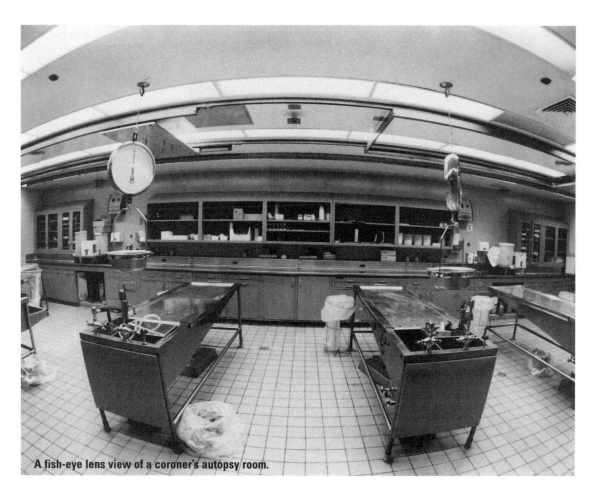
A fish-eye lens view of a coroner's autopsy room.

All the while, there have been investigators in the field, police detectives as well as coroner's investigators. In the television world of *Quincy*, Jack Klugman's character did it all—he was a medical doctor, a coroner, an investigator, and a police detective. Although there was a time when the doctor did visit the scene, that is now in the hands of the trained coroner's investigators. In the real world, the line of demarcation is clear: the police or sheriff's detective is there to find out who did it and why; and the coroner to determine what, how, and when it happened.

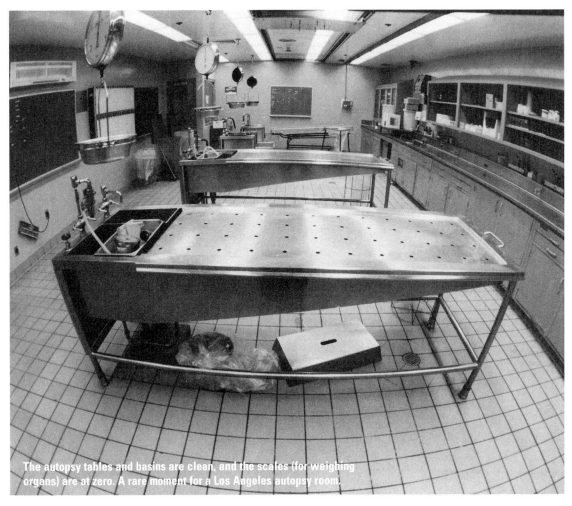
The autopsy tables and basins are clean, and the scales (for weighing organs) are at zero. A rare moment for a Los Angeles autopsy room.

On occasion, the coroner will find overlooked evidence, such as a small fragment of a knife, too small to be detected until a detailed analysis of body parts revealed the fragment. In this case, the coroner becomes a forensic detective, but his evidence is turned over to police detectives so that they can complete their investigations.

Even though *Quincy* distorted the coroner's tasks, it did portray the positive qualities that are an essential aspect of the modern Coroner's Office. It's both the myth and the tales of *noir* that define this jumbled, urban maw.

In L.A., the 20th century has provided so many cases of questionable, high-profile deaths—Marilyn Monroe and Robert F. Kennedy—and lesser-known figures of notorious, unsolved murder cases—William Desmond Taylor, the Black Dahlia, Ronald Goldman. These have seared themselves into the city's collective unconscious.

Raymond Chandler captured the city's off-kilter mood, its endemic corruption, and the "Everyman's" quest to make sense of the mess. Telling Chandler vignettes helped to define the city, with descriptions of landmarks and locales that represent principal *noir* themes: Bay City as political corruption beneath sunshine; Bunker Hill as the decaying heart of the city; Bel Air as *nouveau riche* decadence; Pasadena as old wealth, moral bankruptcy. In this way, Chandler shaped the L.A. persona and lore; and his first novel, *The Big Sleep*, defined the mood later evoked by other *noir*ish film interpretations, such as Robert Towne's *Chinatown*, John Gregory Dunne's *True Confessions*, or the more recent adaptation of James Ellroy's *L.A. Confidential*.

Other great cities of the modern world have their *noir* identities, too; the corruption of New York, Chicago, and Miami; the ghostly spirits of New Orleans; Dashiel Hammett's San Francisco; Paris, Godard's City of Pain; and the celebrated, Victorian mysteries of London. None, though, is so star-crossed as Los Angeles, so littered with celebrity deaths, so filled with irony and contradiction.

Chandler's "Everyman," a lonely figure, fought through the webs of deceit and achieved individual, personal triumphs. This now seems a very distant and romantic vision. No, Los Angeles is now the ideal setting for a *Pulp Fiction*, a series of cruel, irrational, even darkly amusing events, where moral ambiguity reigns supreme, poised on the edge of the unsure millennium to come.

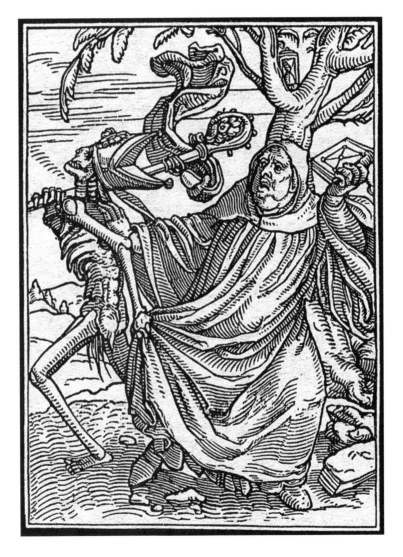

In 1538, Hans Holbein the Younger published his *Dance of Death*, a series of 41 small woodcuts based on the late medieval tradition which gave order and meaning to the inequities of life and to the unexpected (and expected) visitations of death.

The higher one's station in life, the more rudely Death came. For the Abbot (opposite page) and the Abbess (below), Death seizes their robes and deprives them of the relics their profession.

For those who pass through the Coroner's Office, there is no such redress or rationalization; Death is most often cruel and irrational regardless of one's position in this life.

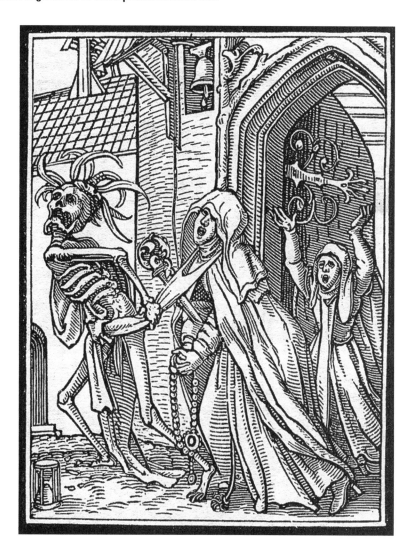

CHAPTER 1

Why the Coroner?

He was smothered . . . his face pressed into the mud. And set afloat in the river afterwards,
With the intent he should be reckoned as one more among the many drowned in Severn.
A mistake! The current cast him up before the river had time to wash away
all the evidences of another manner of death.

—The 12th-century monk Cadfael
from *The Sanctuary Sparrow (The Caedfael Chronicles)* by Ellis Peters

Whenever death strikes suddenly, violently, or unusually, the Los Angeles County Department of Coroner steps in to investigate. Its job is to establish the cause, manner, and circumstances of death, and it has jurisdiction over all homicides, suicides, accidents, and natural deaths when there has been no physician in attendance 20 days prior to the demise. To carry out its mission, the coroner has assembled a team of highly trained investigators, forensic scientists, and pathologists who are supported by skilled forensic technicians, attendants, and clerical staff.

The coroner handles the deaths of people who die on the streets where they sleep. People who die alone, recluses in shabby midtown apartments. People who hang themselves from the balconies of West Valley homes. People who shoot too much heroin or swallow too many pills. People who are stabbed when family arguments turn sour. People who are shot when drug deals go bad. People who are mangled in freeway pileups and crushed when clashing seismic plates make offices and homes crumble.

The L.A. Coroner's Office, the nation's second largest, has never been a typical big-city morgue. Los Angeles County's 4,083 square miles comprise windswept high deserts, sage-walled canyons, a national forest, traffic-clogged urban basins, and beach communities along the Pacific. Over the years, Hollywood has packed the County's refrigerated crypts with world-renowned victims of fortune and fame. Coroner's autopsy tables have cradled the likes of Janis Joplin and Karen Carpenter. Handling Hollywood's famous cases has put the L.A. Coroner's Office prominently in the media spotlight, giving it a strangely glamorous international reputation. In the profession's 800-year history, no other coroner can claim such notoriety.

It all began in the 1850s as a one-man office and grew to today's 180-person operation. Along the way were Wild West killings; Chinatown lynchings; mob violence and murderous union protests; early Hollywood unsolved murders; romantic, ritual suicides off a Pasadena bridge; and a new wave of celebrity deaths after World War II. Its most prominent chief medical examiner, Dr. Thomas Noguchi, was not only a widely admired, pioneering, and skilled pathologist; he was also a celebrity in his own right, the "Coroner to the Stars."

All of this history has fused into L.A.'s paradoxical landscape and become the essential, irrefutable natural history of the place. Through all this, the Coroner's Office, eyes fixed on Paradise's underbelly, has carried out its responsibilities and built on centuries of precedent to create not only the world's most unusual forensic center, but also one of the world's best.

Ancient and Medieval Origins of the Coroner

Since the dawn of civilization, people have struggled to determine the causes of sudden and violent deaths. The origins of forensic medicine—the science of determining the cause, manner, and circumstances of death—can be traced to ancient Egypt, where in 3000 B.C., King Zozer assigned a Chief Justice-Physician to examine suspicious deaths. In the Middle East, pre-Biblical Jewish laws listed the differences between mortal and non-mortal wounds. And in ancient Rome, where the law stressed the importance of medical-legal experts, there were physicians who specialized in diagnosing the causes of unusual deaths. When Julius Caesar was assassinated in 44 B.C., a physician concluded that only one of Caesar's 23 stab wounds was fatal. Several physicians analyzed the body of Germanicus after his suspicious demise in A.D. 19. Debate raged over whether he had been a victim of cardiac arrest or poisoning, and one zealous scholar tried to find the truth by burning the decedent's heart down to ashes.

The first comprehensive textbook on forensic medicine was published in China in 1274. *Hsi Yuan Chi Lu* (*The Washing Away of Unjust Imputations or Wrongs*) detailed how to tell the difference among accidental, suicidal, and homicidal drownings. It also outlined how to use red light, created by holding red silk between the sun and the corpse, to differentiate between bone damage inflicted before and after death.

The actual coroner's profession boasts a colorful history tracing back to a kidnapped king in 12th-century England. In 1192, King Richard the Lion-Hearted was abducted and held for ransom by Austria's King Leopold. The British treasury, however, lacked the funds to meet the ransom demand. To raise money, the Justiciar of England appointed a knight in each shire, or county, to confiscate the property of hanged felons and sell the items of value for the royal coffers. These knights were given the title "crowner," which evolved into "coroner" (a derivative of the Latin "corona," meaning crown).

Over time, the coroners' influence grew. Their primary duties were to keep a record of all criminal activity in their counties, ensure that the local sheriffs collected the royal taxes honestly, and determine the causes of all violent and sudden deaths.

This last task was especially important if suicide was suspected. Medieval English law decreed that a suicide victim's belongings and land be forfeited to the sovereign, and custom dictated the decedent be maligned and buried far beyond the walls of a Christian cemetery. The Church, not to be outdone, condemned the victim's soul to eternal damnation. These indignities could be spared, however, if the coroner decided the self-inflicted death stemmed from insanity or demonic possession. To determine the cause of death, the coroner would inspect the decedent's body for signs that could indicate how he met his demise. If he needed more information, the coroner would hold an inquest, where he would question witnesses and evaluate their testimonies. These early examinations and investigations, though crude by today's standards, spurred the evolution of forensic medicine.

Forensic advances were also occurring on the European continent. In the late 15th century, the Florentine physician Antonio Benivieni performed dozens of autopsies and recorded for the first time how diseased and injured organs lead to untimely deaths. In 1575, the French royal surgeon Ambroise Pare published a guidebook on how to determine if death was caused by lethal wounds, smothering, drowning, poisoning, or lightning. And in 1621, Pope Innocent X's personal physician, Paulo Zacchias, published the first comprehensive study of forensic medicine. Titled *Questiones Medico Regales*, his book analyzed suspicious death cases heard by the papal court.

Another key advancement occurred in 1815, when the Spanish scholar Matthieu Joseph Bonaventura Orfila published a two-volume study of toxicology, the science of determining if chemicals contributed to unnatural deaths. Orfila proposed that in suspected poisoning cases, traces of the lethal toxin could be found in the body's tissues as well as the blood. He worked like a mad scientist to prove it, sometimes boiling whole bodies in vast iron vats.

A few decades later, the technology was developed that could confirm Orfila's theories. In Prague, the Czech physiologist Johannes Purkinje invented an instrument to slice thin, microscopic portions of tissue from internal organs. By placing these slices under a microscope, a physician could study the tissue samples for clues to identify the agent of death. Typically, the way in which the tissues were damaged could reveal if poison, disease, or a foreign object such as a bullet caused the death. This practice was named histology.

Back in England, by the 19th century, the British coroner had evolved into a specialized investigator of suspicious deaths. The profession had gained enough credibility by 1807 for the University of Edinburgh in Scotland to open the world's first department of legal medicine. This is where much of the early groundbreaking research in the "medicolegal" field took place.

In America, the British-style coroner system was adopted as early as the 17th century.

But by the early 1900s, many major cities began changing the way the coroner operated. The traditional layperson investigators were replaced with physicians trained in forensic pathology—the medical specialty of determining cause, manner, and circumstances of death—and laboratories were developed for toxicology and histology. This new approach received a big boost in 1937 when the Harvard Medical School opened the nation's first department of legal medicine.

The Origins of the Autopsy

Literally, "autopsy" means "seeing for oneself." The word combines the Greek prefix "autos" or self and the root "opsis" or sight. When a pathologist performs an autopsy, he or she dissects a dead body to see what caused the death and the pathological changes that brought it about.

The first systematic use of autopsies, however, had nothing to do with determining cause of death. Around 300 B.C., the Greek-ruled city of Alexandria, Egypt, had developed into a world-renowned center for medical reading and research, attracting scholars from around the globe. The Alexandrian attitude stressed using all available means to acquire knowledge, and the young Greek physician Herophilus embraced this approach in his human anatomy research. He became the first person in history to break religious taboos and regularly dissect corpses to explore and document the workings of internal organs. It's reported he was so zealous in his quest to unlock the body's mysteries that he sometimes sliced open the live bodies of convicted criminals.

About 150 B.C., Rome replaced Alexandria as the Western center for medical research, and over the next 300 years, several key advances were made. Through autopsies, it was learned that veins and arteries connected to the heart and that the heart's beating caused the pulse. And for the first time, autopsies were adopted for legal purposes. When Nero, the fifth emperor of Rome, had his mother secretly put to death for criticizing his mistress, he attended the autopsy to ensure authorities found the "correct" cause for her demise.

With the rise of early Christianity, the autopsy fell out of favor, disdained as a desecration of the corpse and prohibited by papal decree for nearly 800 years. But by the 13th century, society recognized the autopsy's importance in determining the causes of suspicious deaths and it was swiftly revived. The Italian professor Mondino de Luzzi at the University of Bologna was considered the leading medieval autopsy surgeon and his textbook *Anathomia*, published in 1487, provided step-by-step methods for internal examinations. *Anathomia* went through 40 editions and remained the standard text through the 16th and l7th centuries, when autopsies were routinely conducted at universities for both anatomical studies and to determine the causes of suspicious deaths.

The foundations of modern autopsy techniques were developed in the 19th century. Carl Rokitansky, a Czech working in Vienna, performed an estimated 30,000 autopsies by the age of 38, and his three-volume instructional text, *Handbuch Der Pathologischen Anatomie*, stressed the methodical examination of damaged organs to help determine cause of death. The most important 19th-century advancement came from the German pathologist Rudolf Virchow, who developed the use of the microscope to study the effects of diseases and injuries upon individual cells.

Today's Methods

Today, L.A. Coroner's investigators respond to the scenes of death whenever police report suspicious or unusual circumstances. While the photographers document the scene, the investigators examine the decedent, interview witnesses, and painstakingly comb the area for clues that may indicate cause of death. Whenever the circumstances require, criminalists, anthropologists, and archeologists may respond to the scene to collect physical evidence and assist with body recovery.

When they finish, the body is removed to the coroner's Forensic Science Center, where it is fingerprinted and prepared for an autopsy or examination. Physical evidence is collected as warranted. Under the direction of the medical examiner (pathologist) who conducts the autopsy, the decedent is photographed and fluoroscoped (x-rayed), and the clothing is evaluated. Then the body's exterior is examined for injuries and identifying characteristics like tattoos and scars. Next, the interior is probed. Various organs are examined for injuries and abnormal findings. Stomach contents are evaluated, and tissue and bone samples are collected, if necessary, and scrutinized with an electron microscope for bullet or knife marks. Samples of blood and other body tissues are collected and sent to the laboratory to be examined for drugs and other toxins. Then the body is sewn up, issued a cause and manner of death, and released to a mortuary of the family's choice.

The coroner issues a final cause of death in deferred cases after the laboratory, autopsy, and investigation results have been combined and analyzed, a process that may take up to two weeks or longer. Occasionally, these efforts fail to clearly determine the cause of death, which is then classified as undetermined. In these cases, the coroner has the authority to conduct a coroner's inquest.

When determining the mode of death, there are times when pathologists lack enough evidence to determine whether the decedent is an accident or suicide victim. In these cases, the coroner may conduct a psychological autopsy. Here, a forensic psychiatrist or psychologist evaluates the victim's mental status in the months prior to death. This may determine whether the decedent was of a state of mind consistent with suicide.

For all autopsied cases, the assigned forensic pathologist prepares a report detailing the cause and mode of the victim's demise. There are five modes: natural, accidental, suicidal, homicide, and undetermined. If it's a homicide, the report is presented to the district attorney, who may request that the medical examiner testify as an expert witness, showing jurors the specific medical and scientific reasons for the decedent's death and how it came about.

From the Investigator to the Pathologist

The point person for the Coroner's Office is the investigator, the first person at the scene of death, whose task is both emotionally and physically demanding, whose role ranges from comforting the grief of family and friends to detailed examination of a body or its partial remains and, finally, to the collection of evidence and even body parts. At present, the Coroner's Office has over two dozen men and women who serve in this capacity.

At the death scene, there is often the overpowering stench of a decomposed body, or a bloody, bullet-riddled corpse. The investigator, hands covered by latex gloves, probes bullet wounds and gaping gashes, and picks up remains from chunks of brain matter to severed body parts and decapitated heads.

The investigators are there not only as professionals dealing with death, but as compassionate individuals who understand that when death occurs, someone must deal with the aftermath. The first step in this process belongs to the investigator, who will provide to the pathologist and the forensics technicians the information and means for determining death.

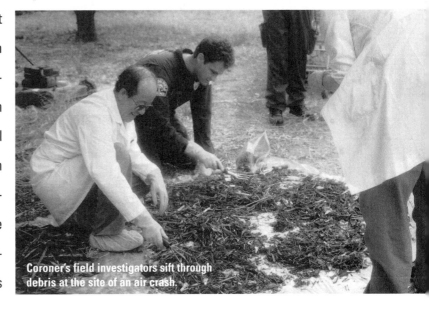
Coroner's field investigators sift through debris at the site of an air crash.

Of the approximately 19,000 coroner's cases each year, slightly less than 10 percent are classified as homicides. For these, the evidence and analysis provided by the investigator and the rest of the Coroner's Office is critical to the police and sheriff's departments' criminal investigations.

In science, one can reproduce experiments *ad infinitum* to confirm results, but this is not a luxury afforded the Coroner's Office. They must carry on their science efficiently and quickly. Once the body and the evidence are in the hands of the pathologist and the forensic technicians, there is seldom a second opportunity to gather more evidence. A

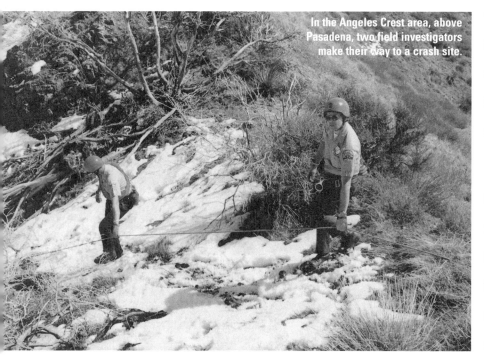

In the Angeles Crest area, above Pasadena, two field investigators make their way to a crash site.

certificate of death needs to be signed— someone needs to put his or her name on the dotted line.

Also, if a case goes to court, the Coroner's representative(s) may be asked unexpected questions, or to certify with exactitude things which cannot always be pre-

cisely determined. For example, if a victim's throat was slashed and the decedent also suffered a blow to the head, it might be hard to assess whether the victim was still alive when the throat was cut. The time of death can sometimes be suggested by tissue damage or other factors, and sometimes this will shed light on the sequence of events. But the Coroner has to withstand speculation, second-guessing, and hindsight from countless quarters, particularly for high-profile cases such as the Marilyn Monroe suicide and the O. J. Simpson trial. For the latter, the more overwhelming the evidence, the greater the potential for nit-picking and for impugning the evidence by way of insubstantial technicalities.

How ironic that the Los Angeles County Coroner's Office has pioneered and expanded investigative techniques and scientific discipline, yet it must deal with outside influences such as the media and the layperson, who are afforded the opportunity to second-guess with the benefit of hindsight—two luxuries denied the coroner and his staff.

How do the investigators, the pathologists, and the forensic researchers deal with the grisly tasks, the damaged bodies, and the grief of those left behind? First of all, they are professionals, and beyond this, in dealing with death, they help bring the tragedy closure. In this process, they are strengthened by their compassion for the families and friends of the victim.

Macabre and seemingly irreverent humor comes into play as well, but this is simply a necessary coping mechanism. Without it, coupled with professionalism and compassion, it would be nearly impossible to handle the relentless stream of evidence, bodies, and grief.

Wild West Roots of the L.A. Coroner

The rate at which people die and how they die can define a region. In 1850, when California joined the Union, "El Pueblo de la Reina de Los Angeles" (the Town of the Queen of the Angels) averaged one homicide per day, making the 4,000-person, tumble-weed town the wildest in the West. On an annual basis, this is 1 in 11 residents; or, in

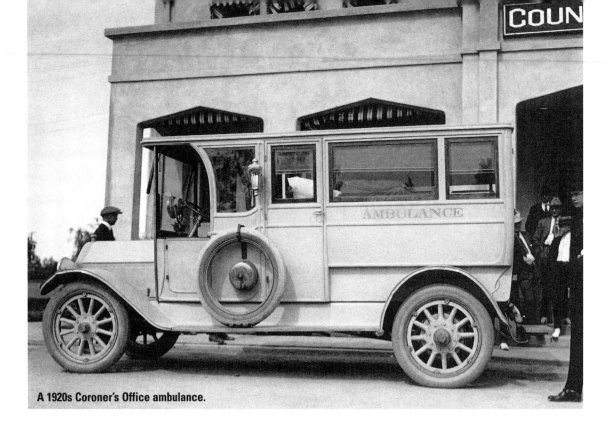

A 1920s Coroner's Office ambulance.

today's terms, for the 134,500 persons in Pasadena, it would be slightly more than 12,000 such cases a year—just for Pasadena.

The newly written California constitution divided the state into 18 counties, requiring each to set up a coroner's office staffed by a single investigator who reported to the county clerk. To determine the cause of death back then, the coroner relied on his deductive skills, but if a case proved particularly complex, he would hold an inquest where, in a courtroom setting, a coroner and jury heard witnesses and defendants testify. The coroner then presented a report of jury's findings to the county clerk.

By the 1920s, the county's population had swollen to over one million, and the eight-man Coroner's Office investigated about 2,500 cases annually.

The Depression fueled suicide cases, including many connected to what became known as "Suicide Bridge." The Colorado Street Bridge, which spans the Arroyo Seco in Pasadena, was the site of 95 suicides, from 1919 to 1937. The most notable of these was the May 1, 1937, death of 22-year-old Myrtle Ward, who threw her three-year-old baby, Jeanette, over the edge and then leapt to her death.

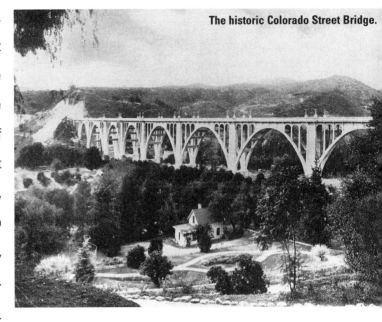

The historic Colorado Street Bridge.

The child landed in some trees, miraculously unscratched. Today, Jeanette Pykkonen is a wife and mother to two girls, living just five miles away from the now-spiked guard rails of Suicide Bridge.

To meet the increasing caseload, the county opened a central Coroner's Office in the Hall of Justice basement located downtown at 211 West Temple Street and expanded the staff to include autopsy surgeons, inquest deputies, deputy coroners, and embalming technicians. Inquests and investigations remained the coroner's main tools to determine cause of death, but as forensic medicine

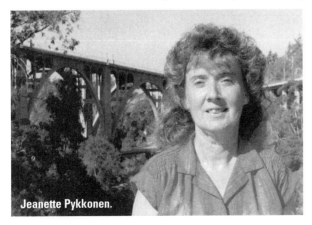

Jeanette Pykkonen.

advanced, autopsies grew in importance, especially in poisonings and drug overdoses.

By the 1940s, with the county population approaching three million, the Coroner's Office saw its caseload top 5,500 per year. It also witnessed a dramatic rise in its use of toxicology. Two forces drove this. First, it was the coroner's task to determine if alcohol was involved in traffic deaths, which climbed rapidly as the use of cars mushroomed. Also, since the coroner resolved whether drug overdoses were accidental or intentional, the office played a key role in determining whether multimillion-dollar life insurance policies had to be paid.

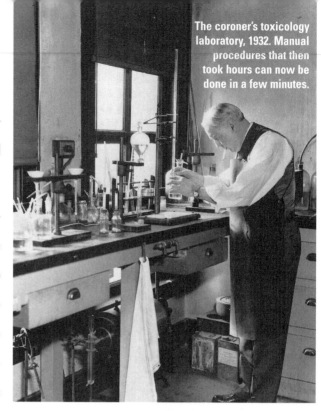

The coroner's toxicology laboratory, 1932. Manual procedures that then took hours can now be done in a few minutes.

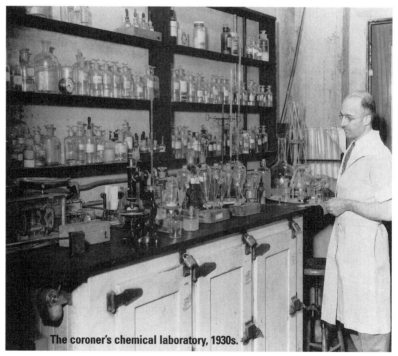

The coroner's chemical laboratory, 1930s.

The Rise of Forensic Science and Medicine

With the explosion of scientific advancements following World War II, the citizens of Los Angeles County voted in 1956 to make the Coroner a medically based institution that specialized in forensic science. The Coroner's Office would be given complete autonomy from the county administrator; it was required by law that this new configuration be led by a forensic pathologist, whose title would be "chief medical examiner-coroner."

Under this system, forensic medicine quickly eclipsed traditional investigations as the primary tool to determine cause of death. And it was L.A.'s first chief medical examiner-coroner, Dr. Theodore J. Curphey, who devised the physiological autopsy, a technique soon adopted throughout the nation.

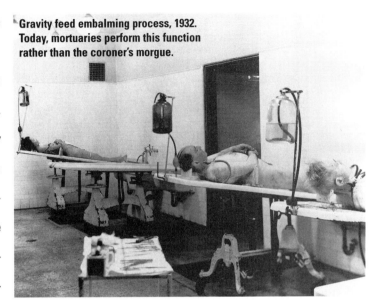

Gravity feed embalming process, 1932. Today, mortuaries perform this function rather than the coroner's morgue.

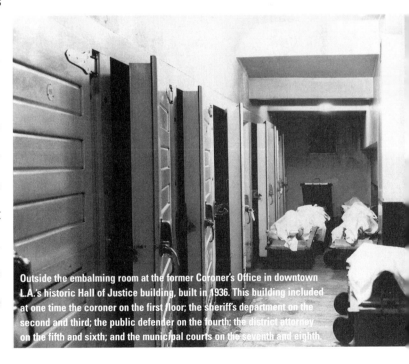

Outside the embalming room at the former Coroner's Office in downtown L.A.'s historic Hall of Justice building, built in 1936. This building included at one time the coroner on the first floor; the sheriff's department on the second and third; the public defender on the fourth; the district attorney on the fifth and sixth; and the municipal courts on the seventh and eighth.

Ironically, the new approach stirred a minor controversy. It became routine for pathologists to take microscopic samples of the decedents' tissues and examine those tissues on laboratory slides. Some religious groups objected, however, arguing that the practice desecrated the corpse and prevented the body from being buried whole. The controversy came to a head in 1959, when the Los Angeles County Board of Supervisors passed an amendment permitting the coroner to retain tissue samples.

In 1965, the position of Coroner's Investigator was created. Working in the field, they serve as the "eyes and ears" for laboratory-bound deputy medical examiners and have proven to be invaluable for local law enforcement.

In the 1970s, two major trends radically altered the way the Coroner's Office did its job. First, the county's population surpassed seven million, and with the crowded conditions, new patterns of death surfaced. The number of drug-related and violent deaths soared, while the Coroner's Office saw its caseload increase to 14,000 annually. This created inevitable backlogs and the need for expanded facilities.

On the flip side, forensic science was booming, fueled by the invention in 1962 of the scanning electron microscope. To exploit this and meet its colossal demand, the Coroner's Office in 1972 moved from its cramped quarters in the Hall of Justice and into the gleaming new Forensic Science Center, a four-story, hospital-sized structure equipped with the latest, cutting-edge technology. The new facility, in the Lincoln Heights district of East Los Angeles, made the Coroner's Office among the most sophisticated in the world and encouraged the development of numerous forensic innovations.

The L.A. Coroner was among the first to adopt the electron microscope for the analysis of gunshot residue and tool marks, compile statistics on cause-of-death trends, and incorporate the expertise of psychiatrists, dentists, and neuropathologists. It also became one of five national centers for training forensic pathologists.

Backed by the center's wealth of technology, the Coroner's Office has helped solve some of the stranger cases to bewilder Los Angeles. One involved two hikers who in 1983 stumbled across a scattering of human bones in the Angeles National Forest. At the Forensic Center, an odontologist x-rayed the jawbone fragments and then matched them with the dental records of a 29-year-old woman who had been missing for eight months. A forensic anthropologist determined that the woman had been stabbed to death, after detecting knife marks on the victim's rib cage.

The next year, in a bizarre case, the Coroner's Office found itself analyzing human bones used in a voodoo ritual. In Marina Del Rey, a boat owner had found a plastic sack of skeletal remains bobbing by his dock. The sheriff's department traced the bag to an elementary school teacher who had purchased a skull, two arm bones, and a leg bone in Haiti from a witch doctor. She had tossed them into the harbor after an argument with her boyfriend, who disapproved of her voodoo rites. But the question remained: Was someone sacrificed for the bones? A Coroner's forensic anthropologist determined that the arm and leg bones belonged to a man, while the skull was that of a 25- to 40-year-old African woman. Lack of evidence precluded a conclusion of murder.

By 1990, however, the Coroner's Office, once again, found its hallways clogged with corpses. The city of L.A. alone fed it several murders a day, while total cases that year reached 18,300.

To improve the management of this torrent of death, the Los Angeles County Board of Supervisors split the Coroner's Office in two. It assigned a nonphysician director to oversee administrative duties, while it made the chief medical examiner-coroner head of the medical staff and responsible for setting standards and

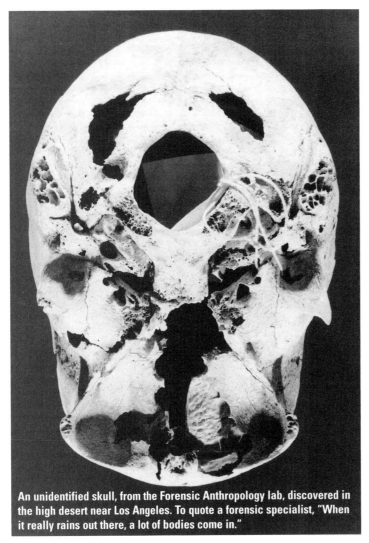

An unidentified skull, from the Forensic Anthropology lab, discovered in the high desert near Los Angeles. To quote a forensic specialist, "When it really rains out there, a lot of bodies come in."

carrying out mandated coroner functions. Both the director and chief medical examiner-coroner are appointed by and report to the Los Angeles County Board of Supervisors. The office was renamed the Los Angeles County Department of Coroner.

Today's department, braced by an $11 million annual budget and 180-person staff, handles more than 19,000 cases a year, the bulk of them natural deaths and accidents. Homicides and suicides account for nearly one-fifth of all cases.

Like the county it serves, the Department of Coroner bustles seven days a week, 24 hours a day, handling a new case every half hour.

It seemed an odd idea, creating an exciting television drama based on the low-profile Los Angeles Coroner's Office. But that's just what NBC did in 1976 when it premiered the hour-long detective series *Quincy*, using

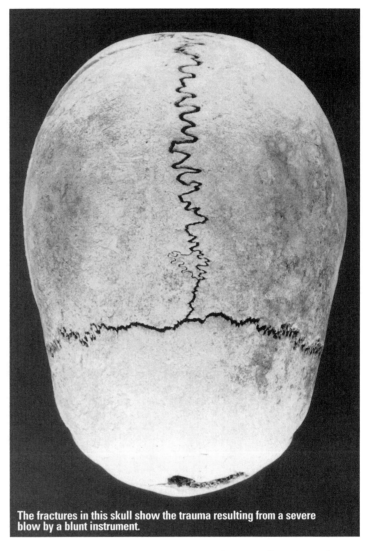

The fractures in this skull show the trauma resulting from a severe blow by a blunt instrument.

members of the Coroner's Office as technical and script consultants. Starring Jack Klugman (known to most as Oscar Madison of *The Odd Couple*) as a crusading medical examiner, *Quincy* was an immediate hit, running for eight seasons and giving the L.A. Coroner international recognition.

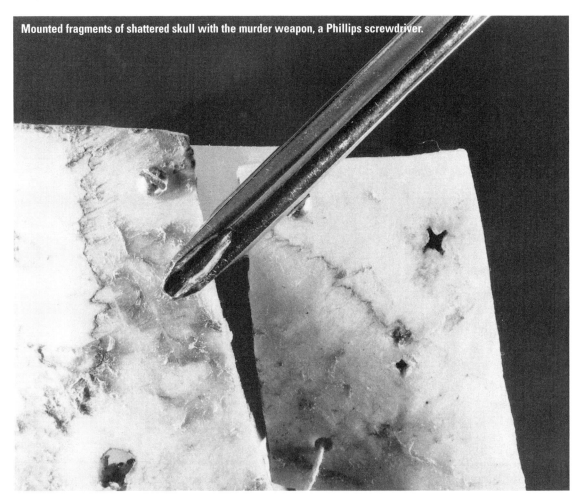
Mounted fragments of shattered skull with the murder weapon, a Phillips screwdriver.

Television audiences quickly took to Klugman's portrayal of a charismatic forensic pathologist with a gruff exterior but a heart always in the right place. Complemented by his refined sidekick Sam (Robert Ito), Quincy hustled around the clock to find the cause, manner, and circumstances of suspicious deaths, even if that meant taking on underworld villains and corrupt politicians.

As Quincy and his team neatly wrapped up the case at the end of each hour, the drama introduced the general public to the difficult issues often faced by medical examiners. In the 1976 opener, "Go Fight City Hall to the Death," Quincy, wielding a flippant, irreverent wit, tackled corruption at the highest levels of L.A. government. Subsequent episodes dealt with rare diseases, autism, the death penalty, medical jurisprudence in rape cases, and, of particular importance to Angelenos, the tragic results of incompetent plastic surgery.

By addressing these issues, the show had an impact that reached far beyond the living room. A 1982 episode, "Give Me Your Weak," dramatized the struggle of "orphan diseases," employing 400 disabled actors to rally for support before a make-believe Congress. Shortly after the show aired, the real U.S. Congress passed the Orphan Drug Act, legislation that gave pharmaceutical companies tax breaks for seeking cures to rare diseases. President Ronald Reagan signed it into law January 5, 1983. That July, the California Governor's Committee for Employment of the Handicapped honored the creators of *Quincy* at its annual media awards banquet.

The present-day Los Angeles County Department of Coroner is far removed from the historical precedents of the coroner, the autopsy, and its own humble beginnings in a sleepy, windswept pueblo. But this history lingers, like faded black-and-white images at the edge of memory.

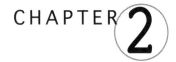

Death in the Pueblo:
Early Coroner's Cases

From the air [L.A.] looks like some enormously exaggerated pueblo itself: flat, sprawling, rectilinearly intersected, dun colored, built of mud brick.... Behind it the tawny mountains run away in a particularly primeval way, a lizardly, spiny way...

—Jan Morris, *Destinations*

When California joined the Union in 1850, Los Angeles was a violent frontier town that averaged one murder a day. Without a railroad, stagecoach, or telegraph link to civilization, this isolated desert outpost attracted a rough, rugged breed of desperadoes, drifters, gamblers, old mountain men, and young fortune hunters. They crammed its saloons and caroused in its plaza, filling the days with impromptu horse racing and the nights with whiskey-fueled mayhem. Ordinary residents strode the streets with revolvers, bowie knives, and rifles.

Most murders took place a block down from the central plaza in a narrow alley called Calle de los Negros (translation: "Nigger Alley"), a cluster of shabby buildings bulging with saloons, bordellos, and gambling dens. After sundown, revelers packed the street, banjo twangs spilled from windows, and gunshots punctuated the air.

The Bella Union Hotel saloon in downtown attracted a hodgepodge clientele, and as the liquor flowed, hotheaded debates raged. One night, a ranch hand named Carlyle flew into a heated dispute with an out-of-town soldier.

"You called me a liar," Carlyle shouted. "Better start shooting." Carlyle drew, but before he could pull the trigger, he took a bullet in the chest. He collapsed, and then, rolling under a table, unleashed a volley of random shots, killing the soldier and two bystanders.

After a trip to this savage outpost in 1864, a startled New York journalist wrote that while sitting at his hotel breakfast table he would "hear the question of going out to

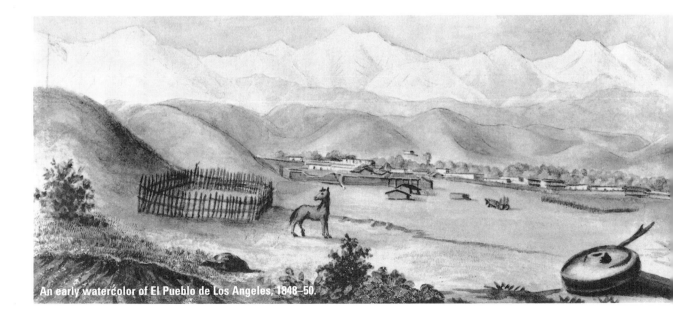

An early watercolor of El Pueblo de Los Angeles, 1848–50.

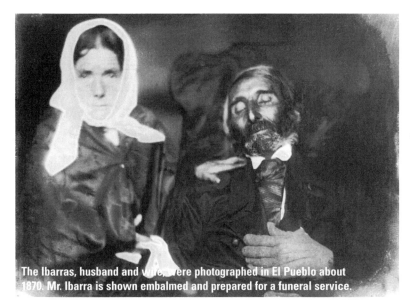

The Ibarras, husband and wife, were photographed in El Pueblo about 1870. Mr. Ibarra is shown embalmed and prepared for a funeral service.

shoot men as commonly discussed as would be duck shooting in any other country. At dinner the question would be, 'Well, how many did they shoot today?'"

Ironically, this rowdy desert town began as a serene Spanish mission.

In 1771, Franciscan friars founded Mission San Gabriel Archangel, an extensive compound where the padres raised cattle, farmed, and upheld Spain's claim to the land. Ten years later, they established El Pueblo de la Reina de Los Angeles as an agricultural supply center for Spanish California. By 1791, the young settlement had a ramshackle central plaza lined with 29 adobe buildings. Its population totaled 139, including 20 families.

By 1822, the year Mexico gained control of California, Los Angeles had evolved into a sleepy hamlet with 2,228 inhabitants. Most residents serviced the wealthy rancheros, whose vast cattle ranches surrounded the town the way suburbs circle the city today.

After the United States seized the California territory in 1847, Los Angeles experienced an economic boom. The gold rush that deluged San Francisco with wealth also funneled fresh capital into Los Angeles. Rancheros saw their profits skyrocket as northern mining towns clamored for Southern California beef, and they lavishly spent their extra dollars in town, constructing churches, opening hotels, and raising stakes at poker tables. The new wealth lured Eastern bankers, Midwestern settlers, and Chinese laborers. It also drew a grim undercurrent of snake oil salesmen.

When the dregs of San Francisco's gold rush community were ousted for any reason, they generally made their way to Los Angeles. Between 1850 and 1870, L.A. became the toughest town in America, averaging a murder a day. It was only appropriate that the City of the Angels was also dubbed "Los Diablos."

The county of Los Angeles in 1850 was then about the size of Ohio, with a total population of 8,300—with 4,000 in El Pueblo. About 71 percent of the county's inhabitants were Hispanic, while Caucasians, Indians, and Asians comprised the rest. That same year, the Los Angeles County legal system was established and Charles B. Cullen was named the county's first coroner. Whenever Cullen felt circumstances surrounding a death warranted an inquest, he was authorized to summon a six-man coroner's jury, and their findings and recommendations were passed on to the county clerk.

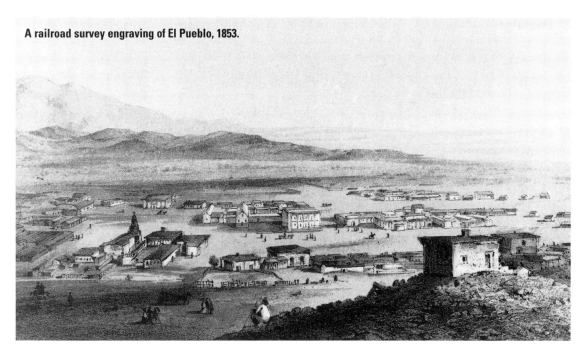

A railroad survey engraving of El Pueblo, 1853.

Early Inquests

In those early years before the railroads arrived, it was rare for a couple of days to pass without a coroner's inquest. In 1850, there were 265. The bulk of them involved deaths in or near the aforementioned slum known as Calle de los Negros, or Nigger Alley (crudely named by the unenlightened in reference to all nonwhites).

The *Los Angeles Star*, the town's first newspaper, would often report the findings. An 1854 article reads, "The coroner's jury sat on the body of a dead Indian. The verdict was: "Death from intoxication."" Another article mentioned that the coroner may examine the death of musician Bass Viol Charlie, who "died very suddenly while playing his favorite instrument at the La Polka Saloon."

There were times when the coroner's findings challenged popular opinion. In 1851, a former Texas cavalry captain named John "Red" Irving galloped into town with a gang of 25 ruffians. When he learned the three sons of the ranchero don Jose del Carmen Lugo had roused the town by murdering two alleged horse thieves, he plotted a way to plunder the Lugo estate. He and his men spread the rumor that the murder victims' kin had formed a posse to exact revenge, hoping the large Lugo clan would temporarily flee their mansion, leaving the valuables unguarded.

But one of the Lugo cousins overheard the plan being discussed in a saloon. And when the Irving gang swept across the Lugo property, Justice of the Peace Jose Maria Lugo and a squad of volunteers ambushed the bandits and slew each one. Although town leaders

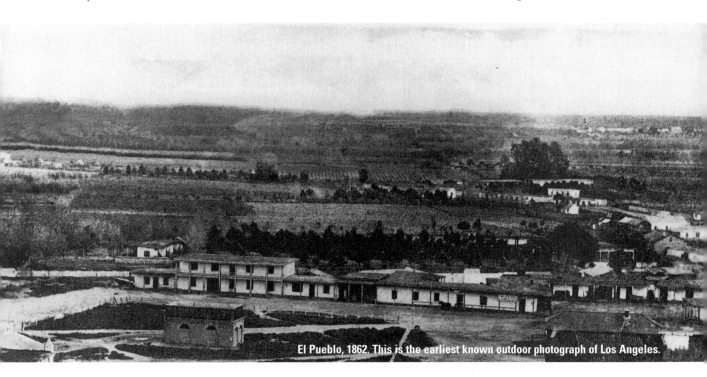

El Pueblo, 1862. This is the earliest known outdoor photograph of Los Angeles.

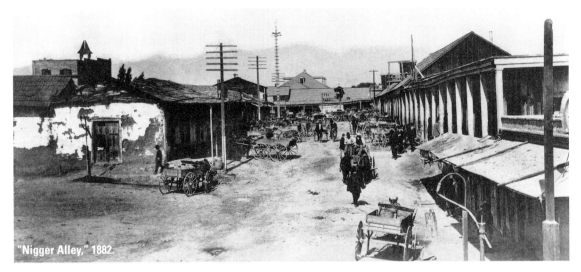
"Nigger Alley," 1882.

questioned the validity of killing all 25 men, most considered the action justified. The coroner's jury, however, found the slaughter excessive, although they conceded the family had the right to protect itself from a band of outlaws who had threatened to "give the Lugos hell." The finding, however, tarnished the family's reputation and led to the demotion of Jose Maria Lugo.

In old Los Angeles, a kind of "lynch law" thrived and often involved its most prominent citizens. Frequently, there was little the legal system, much less the coroner's jury, could do to thwart an angry mob. Indeed, one of the town's most notorious mob murders was led by its mayor.

In October 1854, in broad daylight, the gambler Dave Brown fatally stabbed a cowboy. An outraged crowd grabbed Brown and was preparing a gallows when the mayor, Stephen G. Foster, a Yale graduate, persuaded them to let the courts designate the punishment.

A judge sentenced Brown to be hanged January 12, 1855, but two days before the fateful hour, the state Supreme Court granted Brown a stay of execution. The decision riled the town and an angry throng gathered before the jailhouse. Mayor Foster scrambled atop a beer keg, announced his resignation, and led the horde into the jail. They overpowered the guards, broke into Brown's cell, and dragged the hapless gambler into the street. They hanged him from the crossbeam of a nearby corral gate. When the deed was done, Foster declared himself, once again, mayor.

Tiburcio Vasquez, the legendary bandit who began his career in Northern California, came south to prey on rancheros and stagecoaches in and around Los Angeles in the 1860s and early '70s. Vasquez Rock, off Interstate 14 near Aqua Dulce, about one hour north of Los Angeles, has been the setting for numerous film and television productions. In the 1870s, it was Tiburcio's hideaway.

However, in the next infamous lynching to involve town leaders, the coroner would play a major role in swaying public opinion and bringing justice. One of the town's most dynamic coroners, Dr. Joseph Kurtz, arrived in Los Angeles in 1865 after having served in a Baltimore hospital during the Civil War. German born and educated, Kurtz was a gregarious and convivial surgeon who spent his spare time sipping beer with the other members of L.A.'s Deutscher Klub in a cozy saloon with a sawdust-covered floor and plush armchairs, at the corner of Main and Requena. Later, he became president of the Los Angeles College Clinical Association and in the 1890s played a leading role in the founding of the Medical College of Los Angeles, which would become part of the University of California, Los Angeles.

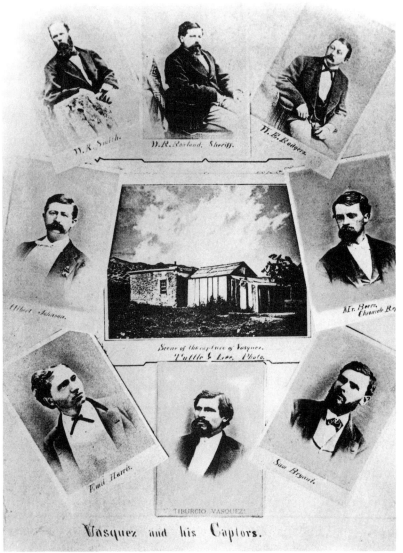

Vasquez and his Captors.

Vasquez's capture in 1874 by Sheriff W. R. Rowland (top center) and his deputies was an early L.A. media event, as shown by this poster.

Legend has it that a botched raid on the Rapetto Ranch (in present-day Montebello) led to Vasquez's capture. Not finding sufficient reward at the ranch, he forced the rancher to sign an $800 check and dispatched a young man to the bank to obtain cash. Suspicions were aroused and a posse followed the messenger.

At first, Vasquez eluded capture and took refuge in the house of Greek George, where he was eventually surrounded. Once in jail, he became a romanticized hero, especially by women, who showered the jail with flowers and gifts. Vasquez, in the end, was returned to San Jose for an earlier crime, and sentenced to hang.

The Chinese Massacre

In October 1871, during his second year as coroner, Dr. Kurtz faced the most formidable task in his medical career. On October 24, a riotous spree ignited on Calle de los Negros and only abated after a mob surrounded the alley and lynched approximately 21 Chinese and looted upwards of $40,000 in gold, jewelry, personal property, and cash from the residents.

Most historians agree a policeman, Officer Bilderain, entered Calle de los Negros to quell a shooting between rival tongs or Chinese communities. He was shot in the shoulder and retreated. A passing rancher, Robert Thompson, sprang to the aid of Bilderain but was shot dead. Another report has Bilderain and Thompson attempting to arrest Sam Yung in his drugstore on Calle de los Negros with a fake warrant, so that they might rob the money in a trunk in the back of the store.

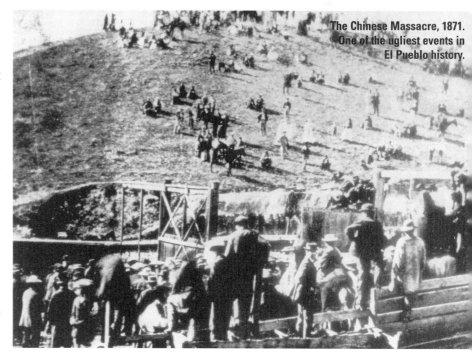

The Chinese Massacre, 1871. One of the ugliest events in El Pueblo history.

In either event, an orgy of violence followed. The police chief ordered his officers to let the mob surge into Chinatown and, according to a number of historians, demanded they shoot fleeing Chinese. Merchants handed out ropes and a city councilman helped determine who was to be hanged. When Dr. Wong Tuck tried to escape, he was grabbed, mugged, and then hanged, but the rope snapped and the mob strung him up a second time, amusing themselves by bashing his head as he dangled from the noose.

The next morning, the corpses, ropes still around their necks, were piled in front of City Hall. But, that same day, Dr. Kurtz ordered 111 witnesses, many of them riot participants, to testify at the inquest. The coroner's jury found that Yung shot Thompson in self-defense, the lynchings were unjustified, and the police were "deplorably inefficient." The coroner's report recommended that the district attorney try 50 of the rioters.

And while the *Los Angeles Star* declared it a "great victory," other journalists were not as jingoistic. The *San Francisco Bulletin* called the Chinese Massacre "one of the most horrible tragedies that ever disgraced any civilized community." East Coast papers were uniformly indignant. The *New York Herald* of October 26 read in part, "The account of Chinese riots in Los Angeles Cal., reads very much like some of the accounts of negro riot in Ku Klux neighborhoods in the South."

Eventually, the Los Angeles City Council paid a substantial indemnity to an outraged China.

Mob rule thrived in old Los Angeles, and, as in the Chinese Massacre, it often involved respected town leaders. Amid this trigger-happy populace, the coroner had to make controversial decisions that often had unforeseen ramifications. One such case involved a duel between Jacob Bell, a wealthy businessman, and Michael Lassanier, a recent French immigrant. Both claimed ownership of 80 acres located where the L.A. Coliseum sits today. The day of the duel, Lassanier and Bell met with a lawyer to resolve the quarrel. "My advice to you," the lawyer said, "is to rely on the law of rifles."

That afternoon, with a single bullet, Lassanier won the land. The next day at the inquest, the coroner determined Bell had fired first and was then killed by a shot to the chest. Since Lassanier fired second, the coroner ruled he shot in self-defense and referred the case to a grand jury.

The self-defense decision riled the town, and that night an angry mob gathered near the jail where Lassanier was held. They ranted, stomped, and shouted, but took no action until a Methodist minister gave a rousing speech, declaring that justice be done. Led by the preacher, the mob burst into the jail, grabbed Lassanier, and paraded him through downtown, seeking an appropriate lynching locale. Surging up Spring Street, the mob found a barrel to use as a hanging platform, and Lassanier soon found himself standing atop it with a noose scraping the skin of his throat. Then, unexpectedly, a young priest jumped up next to him and scolded the mob, shouting that the man they were condemning had "religious privileges."

"Privileges?" yelled Bell's brother. "Let him have 'em in Hell!"

With that, the barrel was kicked over. The priest was knocked to the street, while Lassanier swung from the rope.

In the 1870s, self-defense was reason enough to pull the trigger. Sometimes it was enough to commit what today would be first-degree murder. This was the case when a renowned gunfighter named Joe Dye threatened to kill a Los Angeles deputy sheriff. Dye told the deputy he was heading to Ventura County to work the oil fields, but when he returned, he would hunt him down.

Two years later, the deputy was tipped off that Dye was riding toward L.A., so he and a friend set up an ambush on Commercial Street, downtown. Each positioned himself on opposite sides of the road, the deputy with a rifle in a second-story window, and his partner with a revolver on the street. As Dye swaggered up, he spotted the deputy in the window and drew. But for the first time in his gunfighting career, he fumbled his six-shooter. That gave the deputy enough time to unload three rounds into the gunslinger's torso. At the inquest, the coroner concluded the deputy shot in self-defense and let him go free.

L.A. Times **Bombed!**

Mob rule faded when the railroads arrived. By 1883, both the Southern Pacific and the Santa Fe lines connected Los Angeles to the East Coast. Thousands of newcomers poured into town each year, enticed by ads depicting Los Angeles as a sun-caressed Eden of cheap land and boundless orange groves. By 1888, the tough frontier town had been eclipsed by a vibrant boomtown, with a population topping 40,000, while the county's surpassed 100,000.

As the city expanded, the coroner faced new challenges. Determining the cause of death demanded more sophistication, because the agents of death were no longer limited

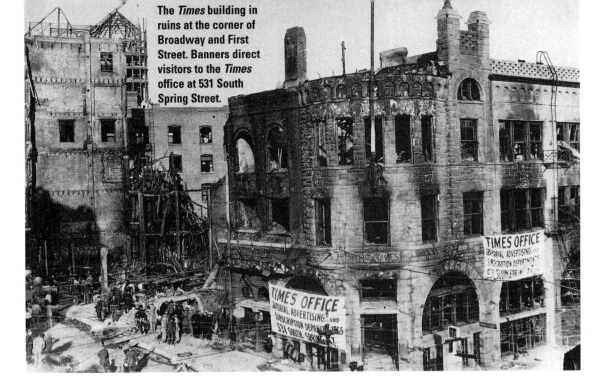

The *Times* building in ruins at the corner of Broadway and First Street. Banners direct visitors to the *Times* office at 531 South Spring Street.

to just bullets, knives, and nooses. The coroner started to conduct autopsies and would call a chemist whenever he suspected poisons or drugs in the blood.

In the newly industrialized city, labor relations became fractious as the downtown power brokers fought to keep the unions out. This struggle climaxed at 1:00 A.M. on October 1, 1910, when a series of explosions ripped through the *Los Angeles Times* printing plant as the

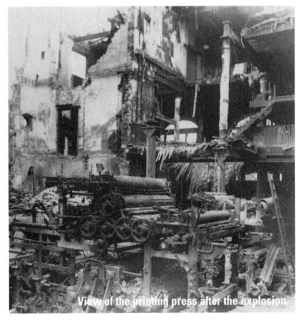

View of the printing press after the explosion.

presses were pumping out the morning edition. The blast blew apart the first floor, and

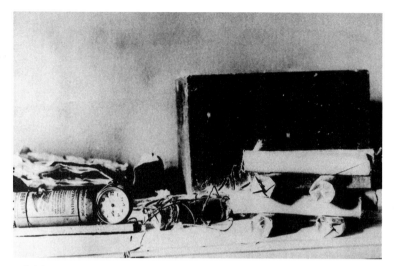

Left: The *Los Angeles Times* bombing was blamed on unionists and there was bad blood all around. This is the bomb found outside the home of and intended to kill Felix Zeehandelaar, an anti-unionist who was secretary of the merchants and manufacturers association.

Opposite: A written confession from one of the McNamara brothers dated December 4, 1911—over one year after the *Los Angeles Times* building explosion.

within seconds, flames engulfed the three-story structure. Only a skeletal building remained when the fire was extinguished. That morning, coroner's deputies raked the ashes to recover the remains of 22 workers.

The *Times* immediately accused union extremists of planting a bomb, while the unions blamed gas leaks from cracked piping. The coroner's inquest, however, found incineration as the cause of death and dynamite the trigger of the flames.

The finding led to one of the 20th century's most notorious trials, with renowned defense attorney Clarence Darrow representing the two suspected bombers, brothers by the name of McNamara. Both sides accused each other of tainting the jury pool and attempting to bribe jurors, while the *Times* published a string of searing anti-union editorials. But four days before opening arguments were to begin, the suspects, on Darrow's advice, pleaded guilty.

Los Angeles Cal
Dec. 4. 1911

I, J. B. McNamara, defendant in the case
of the people against McNamara
and others having heretofore plead
guilty to the crime of murder
desire to make this statement
of facts concerning the same:—
And this is the truth on the night
of ~~Oct~~ Sept 30, 1910, at 5.45 p.m.
I placed in ink alley a portion
of the Times Building a suit case
containing 16 sticks of 80 per cent
Dynimite, set to explode at one o'clock
the next morning it was my intention
to injure the building and scare the
owners. I did not intend to take
the the life of any one. I sincerely
regret that these unfortunate men
lost their lives, if the giving of my
life would bring them back I would
freely give it. In fact to in pleading
gilty to murder in the first degree
I have placed my life in the hands
of the state.

J. B. McNamara

Murder in Old Hollywood

In the early 20th century, a tight clique of Spring Street capitalists controlled Los Angeles's wealth, but in a suburb named Hollywood, there was a fledgling film colony forming, whose power would one day rival that of the downtown establishment.

It began slowly. A trickle of New York filmmakers moved to Los Angeles for the year-round sunshine, then required for filming. They also wished to avoid paying astronomical royalties to Thomas Edison, who held the patent on the motion picture camera and demanded a royalty from every movie made.

The film industry attracted a quirky breed, and even the Los Angeles Coroner's Office, world-weary from decades of Wild West–style murders, was unprepared for the bizarre twists of Hollywood-style death. The first film industry murder still ranks among Hollywood's strangest.

In 1909, director Francis Boggs rented a vacant Chinese laundry downtown at 8th and Olive and converted it into a 40-square-foot stage. There he filmed *The Heart of a Race Horse Tout*, the second motion picture to be produced completely in California.

Boggs then allied himself with fellow director William Selig to make another movie in that space. Apparently, during production, a racket echoed from the building. The clamor irked a Japanese laborer so severely that he barged into the studio and beat Boggs to death. Incidents like that convinced director Cecil B. De Mille to carry a derringer when he came to town in 1913 to film *The Squaw Man*.

Like early Los Angeles, primitive Hollywood attracted a host of cowboys and gun-slingers. Most had abandoned the city by the turn of the century to roam the southwestern plains, but word spread that Hollywood needed stuntmen and $5-a-day extras. Some cowboys never shed their frontier mentality as they swaggered across the studio lots.

When the gunfighter Yakima Jim landed in Hollywood, he spent his days flashing a six-shooter and trying to goad other cowpokes into challenging him. His provocations came to a head when he pulled a knife on Tom Bay, a stuntman and known murderer. Bay yanked out a revolver and filled Jim with lead. The inquest that followed marked the first time in years the coroner had investigated an old-fashioned Wild West gunfight.

Elmer McCurdy: Outlaw, Dummy, and Mummy

In December 1976, a Universal Studios television crew was filming an episode of *The Six Million Dollar Man* at the Nu-Pike Amusement Park in Long Beach. In a darkened area of the park's funhouse, a dummy painted glow-in-the-dark fluorescent red dangled from a makeshift gallows. While a technician was adjusting the dummy for the camera, its right arm fell off. While preparing to glue it back on, he saw

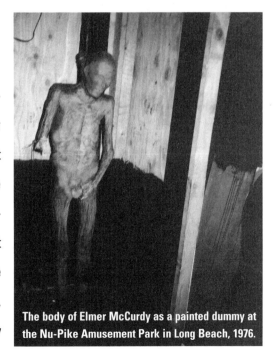

The body of Elmer McCurdy as a painted dummy at the Nu-Pike Amusement Park in Long Beach, 1976.

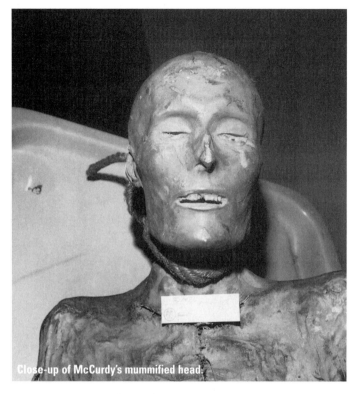
Close-up of McCurdy's mummified head.

what looked like real bones and joints.

A medical examiner from the Los Angeles Coroner's Office confirmed this suspicion. The dummy was actually a mummy.

The next day, a pathologist determined that the rock-hard, paint-covered body was a male Caucasian between 30 and 40 years old. An organic embalming substance had petrified the organs and kept them in their normal anatomical positions. It also seemed a simple autopsy had been performed years ago.

On the chest, a bullet wound was discovered, the projectile's path having ripped through the sixth right rib, the right lung, diaphragm, liver, and intestines. Although the bullet had been removed during the first autopsy, the ballistic configuration of the bullet jacket indicated it had been a .20 to .32 caliber projectile.

Tracing the history of the bullet and embalming substance revealed few clues. The half-copper bullet jacket was introduced about 1905 and discontinued before World War II. The arsenic embalming technique dated back to ancient Egypt, but had fallen out of favor by the early 20th century.

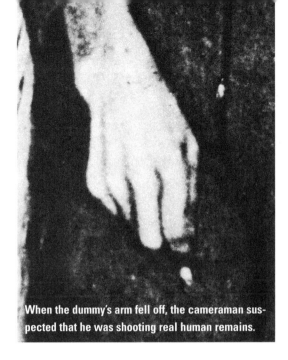

When the dummy's arm fell off, the cameraman suspected that he was shooting real human remains.

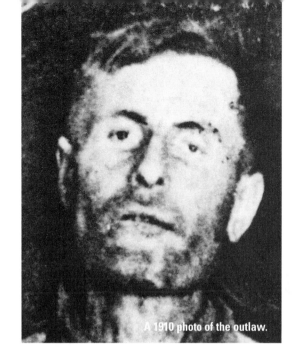

A 1910 photo of the outlaw.

But another examination that turned up a 1924 penny and some old ticket stubs stuffed deep down in the throat helped the Coroner's Office pinpoint the time of death.

Only one ticket stub was still legible. It read "Louis Sonney's Museum of Crime" and listed the address at 521 South Main Street, Los Angeles. Although the museum no longer existed, a Long Beach Police Department detective tracked down the deceased owner's son, Dan Sonney. He recalled that his father had purchased the cadaver of Elmer McCurdy, an Oklahoma outlaw, and kept it in the back of the museum, charging the curious an extra quarter to see it.

Following that tip, the detective learned the outlaw McCurdy had a reputation as an expert safecracker and had allegedly shot and killed a man in Colorado at the turn of the century. Later, McCurdy led various bands of thieves along the Kansas border and served time in the Oklahoma Territorial Penitentiary, from which he escaped. In March 1911, he led an attack on a Missouri Pacific train near Coffeyville, Kansas. That October, he held up a locomotive he thought was carrying thousands of dollars in Indian tribal payments, only to find $46 in the cash box. As consolation, he and his cohorts took off with part of a whiskey shipment. Chased by hounds and a posse, the bandits split up.

Two days later, McCurdy arrived at a ranch in the Osage hills. After drinking with the hands, he was shown a barn to sleep in, but the desperado didn't get much shut-eye. That night, sheriff's deputies surrounded the barn and at dawn demanded he surrender. McCurdy balked and a gun battle raged, ending with the outlaw's death.

The deputies took McCurdy's body to the Johnson Funeral Home in Pawhuska, Oklahoma, but no family ever came to claim it. For four years, it collected dust in a corner. Finally in 1916, two people who claimed to be relatives from California shipped the body out West. After that, it was displayed in nearly every city in the South and the West, eventually ending up at Louis Sonney's Museum of Crime. When Louis Sonney died in 1949, his son put the museum exhibits in storage until 1971 when he sold them to the Hollywood Wax Museum. The museum, however, rejected McCurdy's body, saying it was not "life-like." So the body was sold to the Nu-Pike Amusement Park.

When word spread to Oklahoma that one of their own lay in the L.A. Coroner's Office, they dispatched a forensic anthropologist to California to claim this wayward relic of the Wild West. The anthropologist arrived in L.A. armed with descriptions, mug shots from the old Oklahoma Territorial Penitentiary, and photographs from the University of Oklahoma's Western History collection. The anthropologist confirmed the body was McCurdy's, and it was shipped to Oklahoma in April 1977. Buried in the Summit View

Cemetery at Guthrie, Oklahoma, McCurdy now lies alongside the graves of other notorious outlaws, as well as prominent politicians.

The Baldwin Trunk Murder

While Los Angeles was scandalized by the grisly remains of the Black Dahlia case, to be discussed in the next chapter, it had its predecessor in two 1920s murders where bodies were similarly, unceremoniously dumped. However, these two cases did not go unsolved.

One spring morning in 1924, a matronly, arrogant woman walked into the downtown LAPD headquarters and told the desk sergeant, "Officer, I have killed a man. I want to tell you about it."

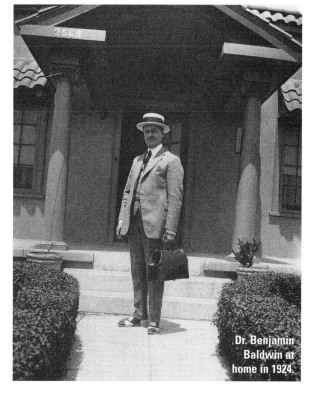

Dr. Benjamin Baldwin at home in 1924.

Mrs. Margaret Willis proceeded to explain that she had shot acquaintance Dr. Benjamin Baldwin as he drunkenly attempted to rape her. She asserted she had stuffed him into a trunk and left him in her apartment for three days, finally dumping it in a remote spot in the hills near San Fernando.

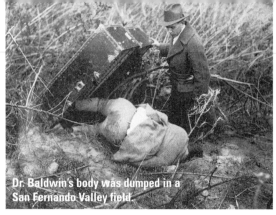
Dr. Baldwin's body was dumped in a San Fernando Valley field.

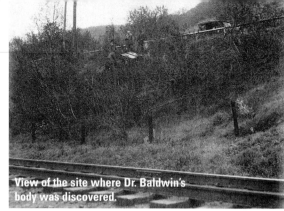
View of the site where Dr. Baldwin's body was discovered.

Sure enough, police found the not-so-good doctor in the now-open trunk among tall weeds, a bullet hole apparent behind his right ear. But even with 1920s rudimentary forensic science, Mrs. Willis's story was found wanting.

The coroner determined there was absolutely no reading for ethanol in the doctor's stomach or brain, disproving her story that he'd been drinking. Furthermore, a large area of powder burns covered the corpse's neck and face, which was not consistent with his being shot up close, during an attempted rape. The shot had to have been fired from several feet away.

Detectives learned that the car in Mrs. Willis's possession, the same used for transporting the body to the hills, was in fact Dr. Baldwin's. Mrs. Willis explained she'd summoned him to her apartment to buy the car for the sum of $700.

But Mrs. Willis's friends confirmed that she was nearly penniless. And then, there was the matter of her having mortgaged the car the day after the killing for $150.

Margaret Willis was tried and convicted of first-degree murder. At the time, women convicts were not hanged, so she was given the rest of her life behind bars to contemplate how she might have better planned the Baldwin Trunk Murder.

After "The Fox"

The 1920s in Los Angeles could still have been characterized as the Wild West. And no case caused as much fear and revulsion among the populace as the kidnapping and murder of 12-year-old Marion Parker in 1927. The action was brutish; the ransom negligible; and the perpetrator completely atypical, a former high school scholastic star named William Edward Hickman.

It began with a "well dressed, nice-looking" man entering the registrar's office at Mt. Vernon Junior High School. He explained his employer, banker Perry Parker, had been in an auto accident and wanted his "younger" daughter by his bedside. Marion was summoned and left with Hickman. It was five minutes after they left that the registrar thought it strange that Parker had twin daughters and only wished to see one.

A telegram that afternoon was followed by a letter the next day, demanding the relatively small sum of $1,500. The same day, a more menacing letter arrived: "Get this straight. Your daughter's life hangs by a thread and I have a Gillette ready and able to handle the situation...Do you want the girl or the 75 $20 gold certificates? You can't have both and there's no other way out..." It was signed, "FOX–FATE."

That evening, the phone rang at the Parker house. After a moment of silence, a voice said, "I am the Fox. Have you got the money?" Parker said he did and the voice replied, "Give me your word as a Christian gentleman you will not try to trap me." Parker gave no answer, knowing that the LAPD had promised to apprehend him.

The meeting that night at 10th and Gramercy was thoroughly botched by the LAPD's

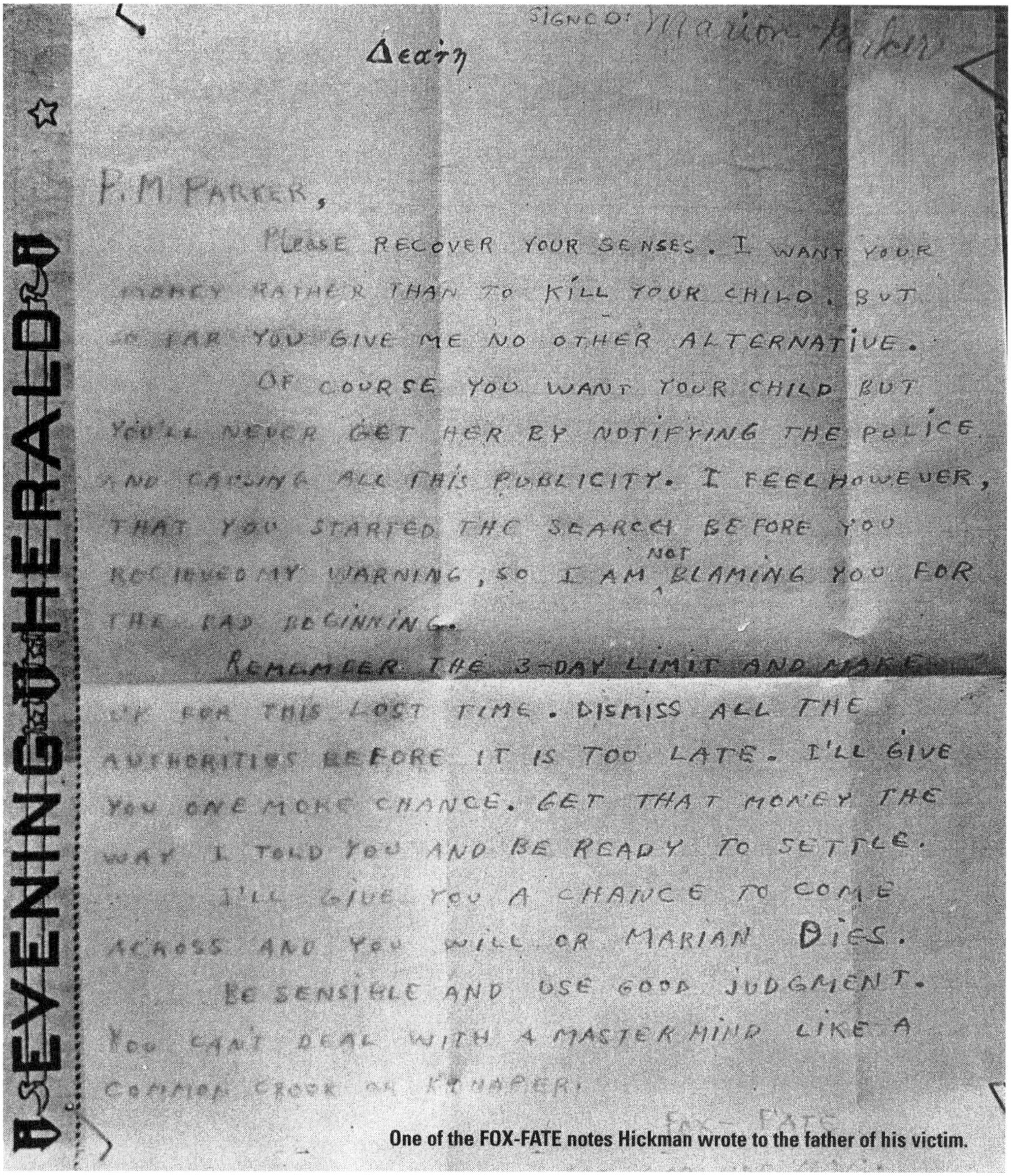

death

SIGNED: Marion Parker

P. M. PARKER,

PLEASE RECOVER YOUR SENSES. I WANT YOUR MONEY RATHER THAN TO KILL YOUR CHILD, BUT SO FAR YOU GIVE ME NO OTHER ALTERNATIVE.

OF COURSE YOU WANT YOUR CHILD BUT YOU'LL NEVER GET HER BY NOTIFYING THE POLICE AND CAUSING ALL THIS PUBLICITY. I FEEL HOWEVER, THAT YOU STARTED THE SEARCH BEFORE YOU RECEIVED MY WARNING, SO I AM NOT BLAMING YOU FOR THE BAD BEGINNING.

REMEMBER THE 3-DAY LIMIT AND MAKE UP FOR THIS LOST TIME. DISMISS ALL THE AUTHORITIES BEFORE IT IS TOO LATE. I'LL GIVE YOU ONE MORE CHANCE. GET THAT MONEY THE WAY I TOLD YOU AND BE READY TO SETTLE.

I'LL GIVE YOU A CHANCE TO COME ACROSS AND YOU WILL OR MARIAN DIES.

BE SENSIBLE AND USE GOOD JUDGMENT. YOU CAN'T DEAL WITH A MASTER MIND LIKE A COMMON CROOK OR KIDNAPER.

FOX—FATE

One of the FOX-FATE notes Hickman wrote to the father of his victim.

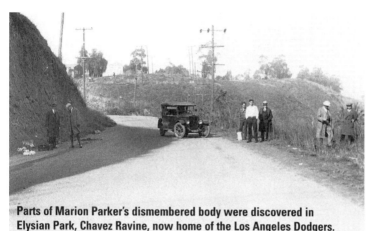
Parts of Marion Parker's dismembered body were discovered in Elysian Park, Chavez Ravine, now home of the Los Angeles Dodgers.

obvious stakeout of the entire neighborhood. Hickman saw the squad cars and drove back to his dingy apartment, while Marion sat next to him, sobbing quietly.

That night, Hickman strangled Marion Parker to death with a towel as she sat bound to a chair. But in his letter the next day to Parker, Hickman wrote: "You are insane to betray the love of your own daughter..." He offered to meet Parker that evening, a supposed last chance.

At eight o'clock, Parker drove to an address in the Wilshire district, parked, and waited. The dark street was deserted. Within minutes, a car with its headlights off pulled up alongside him. The driver was pointing a shotgun at him. The dark outline of Marion's profile was barely visible.

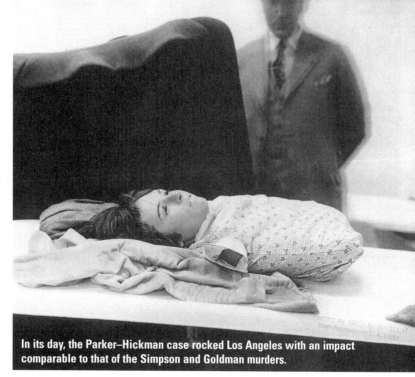
In its day, the Parker–Hickman case rocked Los Angeles with an impact comparable to that of the Simpson and Goldman murders.

"I am the Fox," said the driver. "Hand me the money." Parker tossed the bundle. "Don't follow me" was the driver's response.

Parker watched as his tormentor drove to the corner, stopped, left something on the curb and drove off. Parker drove quickly to the site and withdrew a blanket covering Marion's butchered torso, the lifeless, frozen face staring upward, two long, black threads pierced through each eyelid, holding them open.

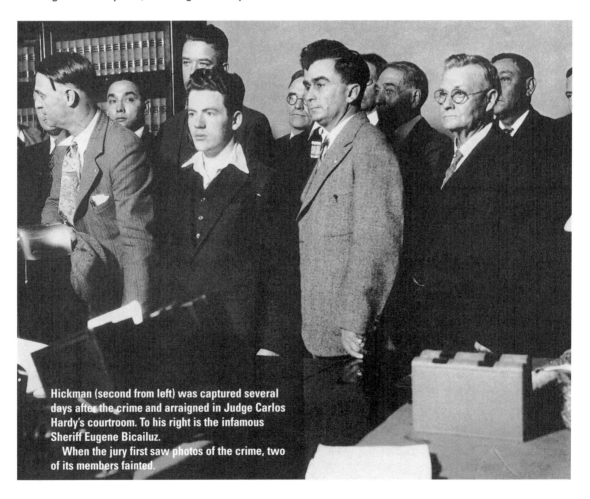

Hickman (second from left) was captured several days after the crime and arraigned in Judge Carlos Hardy's courtroom. To his right is the infamous Sheriff Eugene Bicailuz.

When the jury first saw photos of the crime, two of its members fainted.

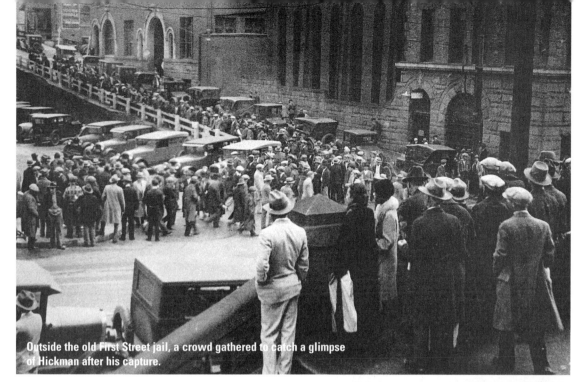

Outside the old First Street jail, a crowd gathered to catch a glimpse of Hickman after his capture.

Hickman was caught days later. He was tried, found guilty, and hanged.

In the first hours of the Parker–Hickman case, young men who remotely fit Hickman's description had been arrested, even beaten by irate mobs, shocked by the act perpetrated against a defenseless young girl. One suspect bore such a strong resemblance to Hickman, he was arrested twice. The attendant notoriety led the man to commit suicide.

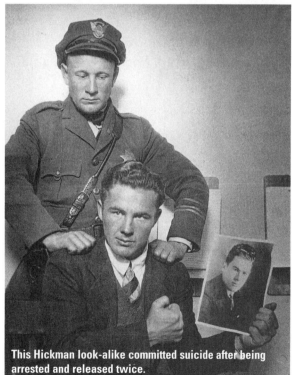

This Hickman look-alike committed suicide after being arrested and released twice.

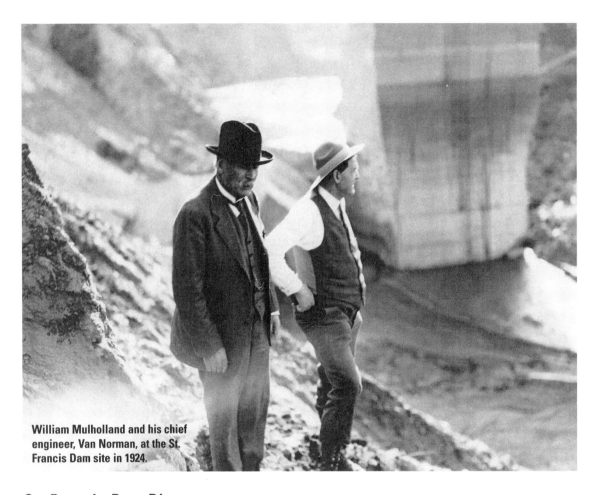

William Mulholland and his chief
engineer, Van Norman, at the St.
Francis Dam site in 1924.

St. Francis Dam Disaster

William Mulholland's surname is synonymous with the picturesque drive that winds
through the Hollywood Hills, reaching to the San Fernando Valley. Yet what should have
been the crowning achievement of his life, the 1924 completion of the St. Francis Dam
near Castaic, resulted in a tragedy that equaled the better-known San Francisco earthquake of 1906.

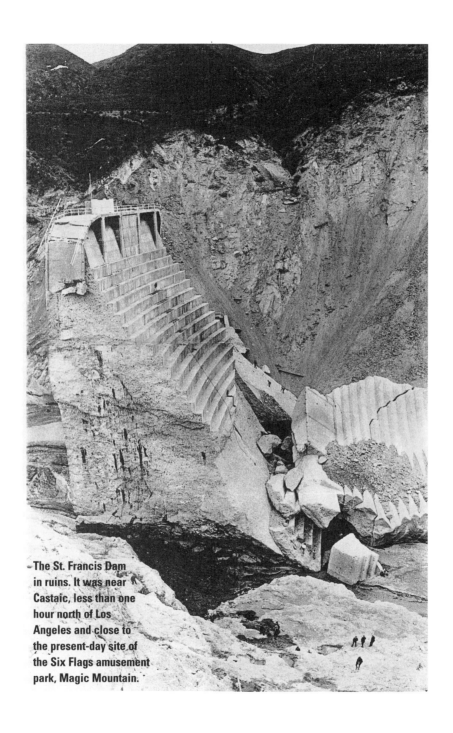

The St. Francis Dam
in ruins. It was near
Castaic, less than one
hour north of Los
Angeles and close to
the present-day site of
the Six Flags amusement
park, Magic Mountain.

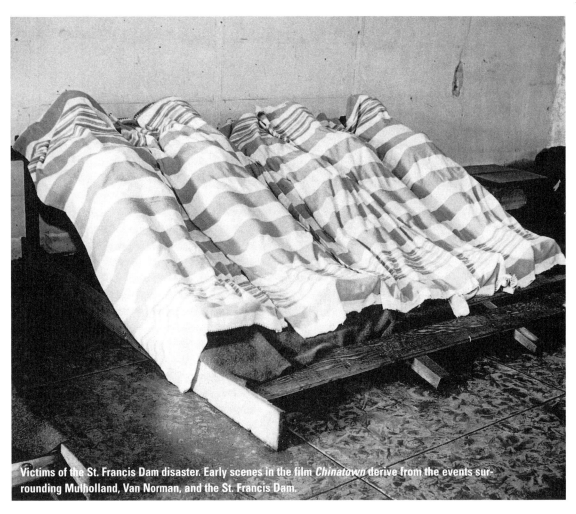

Victims of the St. Francis Dam disaster. Early scenes in the film *Chinatown* derive from the events surrounding Mulholland, Van Norman, and the St. Francis Dam.

Having arranged, via underhanded means, to siphon the water from the ranchers of the Owens Valley, Mulholland, aided by chief engineer Van Norman, constructed the St. Francis Dam, fed by the Owens Valley Aqueduct, 250 miles of pipes, tunnel, and concrete. The dam itself was as tall as an 18-story building at 185 feet, with a powerhouse control room that harnessed a steady flow of 50,000 kilowatts of electricity.

But on March 12, 1928, the 12 billion gallons of water it held burst forth, after a collapse that, to this day, cannot be fully explained.

The official story was that the west wall of the San Francisquito Canyon became saturated and gave way under the weight of the dam. But despite the 850 pages of testimony in the coroner's inquest that came later that month, rumors still swirled that angry Owens Valley ranchers had dynamited the dam. Had a previous landslide on the east end of the canyon had anything to do with it? The dam keeper had dug steps up the canyon wall as a possible escape route and no one could explain how the body of his mistress ended up at the base of the dam, upstream from the house where she should have been sleeping.

William Mulholland, father of Los Angeles's water system, who had inspected the dam just hours before, saw his status, and hopes for a political career, washed away, along with the lives of 450 people.

CHAPTER 3

A Star-Studded Caseload

And since Sebastian counted among the intruders his own conscience and all claims of human affection, his days in Arcadia were numbered.... He did not fail in love, but he lost the joy of it.

—Evelyn Waugh, *Brideshead Revisited*

Unlike other counties, the coroner in Los Angeles must deal with cases involving that peculiar, fascinating realm known as Hollywood, where ego, sensitivity, power, and highly unique pressures often combine to create high-profile instances of suicide, accidental death, and homicide. Some of these cases are straightforward, noteworthy for their historical precedent, while others continue to baffle us, perhaps forever, for their mystery and lack of closure.

Barbara La Marr

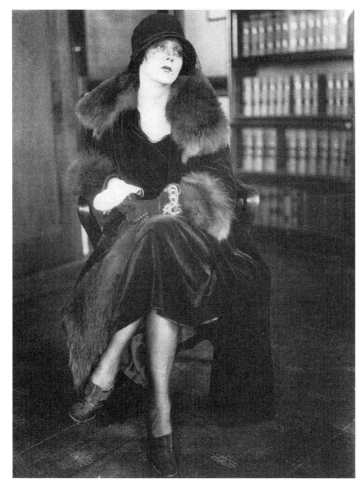

The 1920s may have been considered Hollywood's Golden Age, but to the Coroner's Office, the decade ranks among the film industry's deadliest. Drug abuse put numerous showbiz denizens atop the autopsy tables. Few understood the consequences of chronically consuming cocaine and opium, two drugs which had been legally available on pharmacists' shelves only the decade before.

Barbara La Marr was, then, filmdom's femme fatale. The traffic-stopping star of *Souls for Sale*, *Strangers of the Night*, and *The Heart of a Siren* lived more indulgently than the characters she portrayed. She had dozens of lovers, married five times (first at the age of 16), smoked high-grade opium, and kept her cocaine in a golden casket atop a grand piano.

La Marr's friends fretted over the actress's self-destructive ways, and they were right

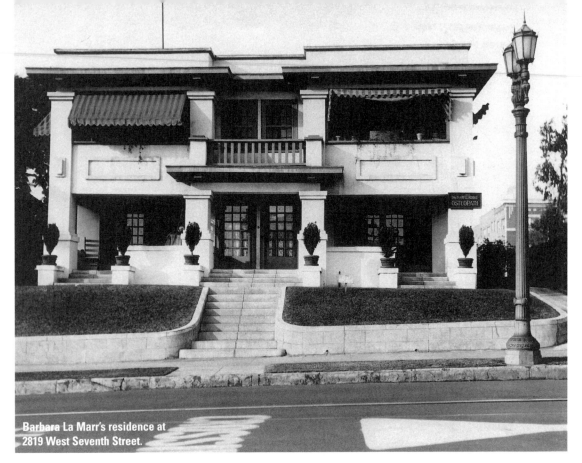
Barbara La Marr's residence at
2819 West Seventh Street.

to do so. La Marr had been born Rheatha Watson. But, depending on whose records you believed, she was born July 28, in either Richmond, Virginia, or Yakima, Washington. The year was a choice of either 1896 or 1900.

In fact, record keeping was not the strong suit of the age. The Coroner's Office used what was called a "Coroner's Register," a simple two-page form which listed the name and age of the deceased, address, and names of those doctors and investigators involved the case. If cause of death was readily apparent, it would also be listed as well.

La Marr drank too much; gained weight, then crash-dieted; neglected her work, then suffered the emotional consequences. She became seriously ill in New York and while at the Altadena home of star Zasu Pitts, La Marr succumbed to narcotics. However, the press euphemistically reported that she died as a result of "overdieting."

In marked contrast to coverage of high-profile deaths in current society, the *Illustrated Daily News* of January 31, 1926, took a soft approach to her continuing addiction, eulogizing, "The famous vampire of the screen lost her long fight."

Befittingly, Barbara La Marr had been known throughout her tumultuous career as "the girl who was too beautiful."

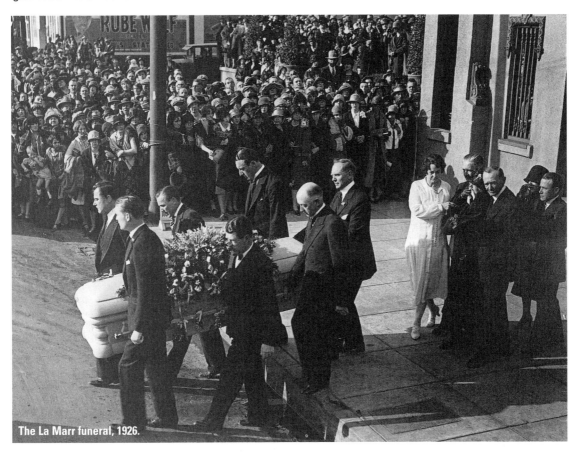

The La Marr funeral, 1926.

William Desmond Taylor

In 1922, this 45-year-old former bit player had become Paramount Pictures' leading director, when one of Hollywood's most complex and fascinating unsolved murder mysteries transpired.

The form found in Coroner's Office files listed Taylor's date of death as February 1, 1922, and the declarative statement from a jury: "Gunshot wound of the chest inflicted by some person or persons unknown to this jury, with intent to kill or murder."

The story, while convoluted, is the stuff of legends. In 1908, a struggling Irish actor named William Cunningham Deane-Tanner, comfortably situated with family and antiques store, began stumbling home drunk, often reeking with the sex of other women. One morning, he telephoned his store to demand $500 be wired to a Manhattan hotel. After receiving the money, he vanished.

Five years later, a charming thespian named William Desmond Taylor appeared in Hollywood, strutting about in a British Army officer's uniform, boasting of military feats, landing a string of acting jobs. In 1916, having directed a number of minor flicks, Taylor became a director for Paramount Pictures and carved his niche as a maker of family films, directing *Tom Sawyer*, *Anne of Green Gables*, and others. He worked with some of America's most beloved stars, including Mary Pickford and Mary Miles Minter, both adored for their demure innocence, girlish curls, and cherubic smiles.

Gossip circulated that the single gentleman was gay, a rumor that grew when Taylor hired an effeminate, soprano-voiced male butler who had been arrested for soliciting boys in Westlake Park. Busybodies also wondered why Taylor had abruptly fired his valet, Edward Sands, insinuating that something darker lay beneath the allegations of check forgery and petty theft.

Taylor, who resided in a fashionable garden court bungalow at 404 B Alvarado Street, spent the evening of November 1, 1922, entertaining the comedic star Mabel Normand, a 28-year-old whose slapstick finesse brought fame to the Keystone Kops.

Within 30 minutes of Normand's departure, however, an overcoated figure with a hat pulled low, a muffler over the mouth, and a .38 caliber revolver in hand crept into the bungalow and unloaded a single round into the director's back.

Around 7:30 the next morning, the butler discovered his employer laying in a puddle of coagulated blood. Frantic, he scampered down Alvarado Street, shrieking that his master had been iced. The screams woke actress-neighbor Edna Purviance (noted for her work in Charlie Chaplin's films). She rushed next door to find Taylor, dashed

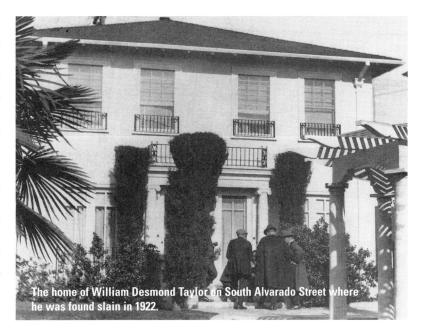

The home of William Desmond Taylor on South Alvarado Street where he was found slain in 1922.

home and phoned Normand, then placed a call to Paramount Pictures and another to the mother of Mary Miles Minter.

By the time the police arrived, Normand was rifling through the closet. Paramount mogul Adolph Zukor himself was tossing sheets of paper into a blazing fireplace and his second-in-command, Charles Eyton, was gathering bottles of bootleg booze. And a quivering Edna Purviance, white as a ghost, stood stiff against the wall.

In minutes, a detective squad descended, befuddled to find so many people milling about the deceased. Then a middle-aged man lumbered into the confusion, proclaimed himself a doctor, and declared the deceased a victim of a stomach hemorrhage triggered by natural causes. Within an hour, as the coroner's ambulance arrived, the investigators were preparing to close the case. But as the coroner's attendant lifted the corpse onto the gurney, the detectives spotted the bullet hole in its back. The investigators herded everyone outside and began conducting interviews for a murder investigation. They combed the area for the alleged doctor, but he had vanished.

They did, however, find a witness. From her courtyard window, Faith Cole MacLean, wife of actor Douglas MacLean, told officers she had heard a "small explosion" and then saw a figure in overcoat, cap, and muffler scurrying from Taylor's bungalow. It was dressed like a man, she said, but "…it walked like a woman, quick little steps and broad hips and short legs."

Two days later at the coroner's inquest, it became clear the distinguished director had lived a double life. In his bungalow, detectives had found a cache of pornographic photos

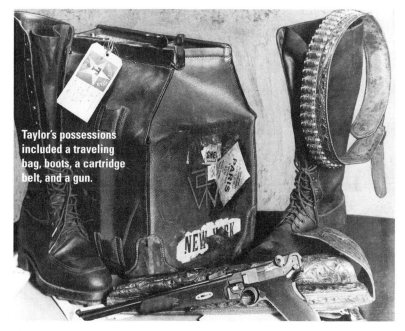

Taylor's possessions included a traveling bag, boots, a cartridge belt, and a gun.

of Taylor and numerous, well-known screen beauties. In his riding boots, they uncovered a bundle of love letters from Mabel Normand. In the bedroom closet, they came across a collection of women's underwear, each tagged with its owner's initials and the date of conquest. Among them were a pair of pink, French-made panties embossed with the initials MMM.

A 22-year-old Mary Miles Minter claimed innocence, but when strands of her hair were uncovered in the bungalow, it became impossible to deny that Minter, the virginal screen princess, had been Taylor's lover. At the time of his murder, police concluded, Taylor was having simultaneous affairs with Normand and Minter. They also suspected he was sleeping with Minter's mother and the screenwriter Zelda Crosby, who committed suicide after the funeral.

For months, investigators hounded Normand, but then dismissed her as a suspect. The investigation of Minter, however, destroyed the young actress's career. Driven by an obsessive showbiz mom, Minter was legally obliged by the Paramount brass to uphold her pure image off-screen and remain unmarried. Minter made six films after Taylor's death,

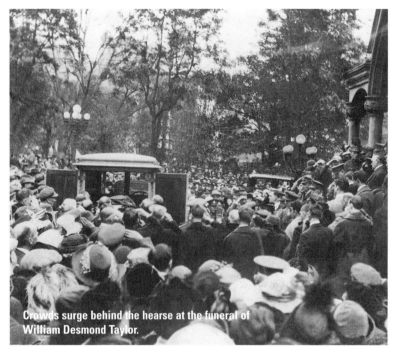
Crowds surge behind the hearse at the funeral of William Desmond Taylor.

but Paramount refused to release them. Defeated, she and her mother withdrew to a Santa Monica cottage, where the shapely Minter ballooned into obesity by gorging her sorrows away with chocolate.

Within six weeks of the homicide, 300 people confessed to the killing, although none could provide evidence supporting his or her macabre claim. A drug angle did emerge when a tipster claimed to have heard Taylor, on the night before his murder, arguing with a bootlegger who supplied drugs and booze to the film community.

It didn't surprise Tinseltown when detectives discovered Taylor frequented shadowy dens that served opium, cocaine, and marijuana. They shrugged when newshounds reported Taylor was often seen with a pusher on the studio lots and that he had ties to two elusive morphine dealers. But jaws did drop when police unearthed a blackmail motive.

Apparently, Normand snorted $2,000 of coke each month, and Taylor helped procure the needed supply. Police believed one of Normand's dealers may have boosted his income by blackmailing her. Witnesses reported seeing Taylor approach this particular pusher and pound him to the sidewalk with a volley of hooks and jabs.

Like the other leads, however, the drug angle fizzled. It was, though, soon replaced by the strangest twist yet. Investigators traced Taylor's path back to the New York antique store and a small town in County Cork, Ireland. That's when they learned Taylor's valet was actually his younger brother, Denis Deane-Tanner. Police figured he may have fired the deadly bullet, motivated by rage after being fired.

Apparently, the younger sibling had come to L.A. after committing a string of burglaries on the East Coast, leaving behind a wife and two children. In Hollywood, he had dyed his hair blond, assumed a servant's deferential pose, and joined his elder kinsman in sexual adventures. Denis was believed to have taken all the photographs in Taylor's porn collection. But when efforts to find him failed, the LAPD suddenly closed the case, labeling it "unsolved."

No one understood why the police, for two years hell-bent on solving the crime, turned their backs. It's alleged, however, that studio honchos cut a deal to halt the investigation, and its attendant bad press, with Los Angeles District Attorney Thomas Lee Woolwine.

It's also reported that Hollywood insiders knew the murderer's identity: Charlotte Shelby, mother of Mary Miles Minter. After learning Taylor had deflowered her daughter, the rumor went, Shelby, herself obsessed with Taylor, had unleashed her vengeance.

The *Los Angeles Herald*'s Hollywood beat reporter, Adela Rogers St. John, was convinced Shelby had pulled the trigger. Shelby fit the sole witness's description of a figure with broad hips and short legs. She also owned a .38 caliber pistol and had been seen practicing at shooting ranges in the months before the homicide. St. John even asked Woolwine why he didn't arrest the person who "…you know did shoot Taylor."

According to St. John, the D.A. guiltily responded, "You know I couldn't convict her."

Peg Entwhistle

In the 1930s, the Coroner's Office faced a new morbid trend—distraught actresses leaping to their deaths from the HOLLYWOOD sign, which then read HOLLYWOODLAND, towering over the real estate development of the same name. The macabre fad was started by Peg Entwhistle, a successful stage actress who tried unsuccessfully to break into the movies.

The Coroner's Register lists Lillian Millicent Entwhistle as "24 years, 7 months, 12 days" of age, when her body was found September 18, 1932, two and a half miles northwest of the end of Beachwood Drive, the street that leads to the sign. It was a warm night when Entwhistle leapt from the 50-foot-high H of the sign. The next day, a hiker on a nearby trail found her body, as well as shoes, jacket, purse, and a note that read, "I am afraid I am a coward. I am sorry for everything. If I had done this a long time ago, it would have saved a lot of pain."

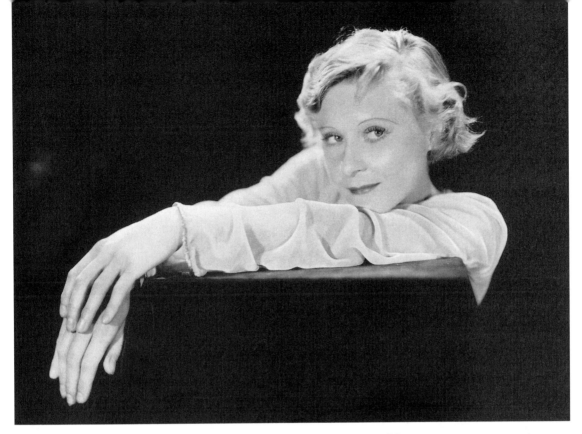

In reality, Entwhistle had the courage to leave London and her stage parents at the age of 14, to chart her career in Boston, then New York City, where she appeared in eight plays. In 1931, she had come to Hollywood and the waiflike blonde's only role, in the film *Thirteen Women*, was virtually eliminated in the editing room.

The 24-year-old actress had stayed with her uncle Harold at 2428 Beachwood Drive. On her last day, she wore a dress she had bought because it belonged to an admired silent-film star. In order not to create suspicion, she told her uncle she was going out to buy some cigarettes.

The Coroner's Register listed a "y.m. [yellow metal] breast pin," which was delivered, postmortem, to Entwhistle's uncle. In typical, bureaucratic language, the report cited "Multiple fracture of the pelvis. Suicidal. Jumped from sign." Yet, when it came to describing probable cause of death, the Register used a single, powerful word which aptly summarized Entwhistle and those who would follow her tragic path: "despondency."

In one of the most vicious twists of Hollywood fate ever, a letter from the Beverly Hills Playhouse was mailed to Peg Entwhistle the day before her fatal leap. Its contents: the offer of the lead role in a play—about a young woman driven to suicide.

Thelma Todd

The decade's most renowned Coroner's Office case, however, involved one of the decade's most successful actresses. A wisecracking, blonde bombshell, Thelma Todd excelled at a bawdy brand of slapstick that made her a favored leading lady in Marx Brothers and Laurel and Hardy films. At 29, the former Massachusetts schoolteacher was enjoying all the frills of celebrity. She lived with ex-film director–producer Roland West and they opened a very successful cafe named Thelma Todd's Roadside Rest, which drew a swanky film industry clientele.

It all collapsed early Sunday morning, December 16, 1935, when she was found dead in her car in the garage she shared with West, enveloped in a cloud of car exhaust. The autopsy report, written by surgeon A. F. Wagner, found Todd's blood "to contain 75 to 80% carbon monoxide saturation." Her brain tissue had only 0.13 percent ethanol, which suggested she was not very intoxicated. There were drops of blood in her nose when maid May Whitehead found her, slumped over, door open, the engine of her powerful 12-cylinder Lincoln still running.

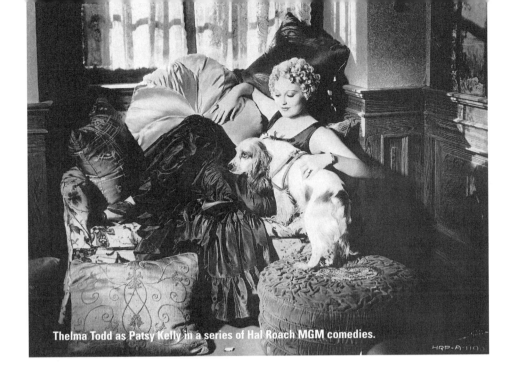

Thelma Todd as Patsy Kelly in a series of Hal Roach MGM comedies.

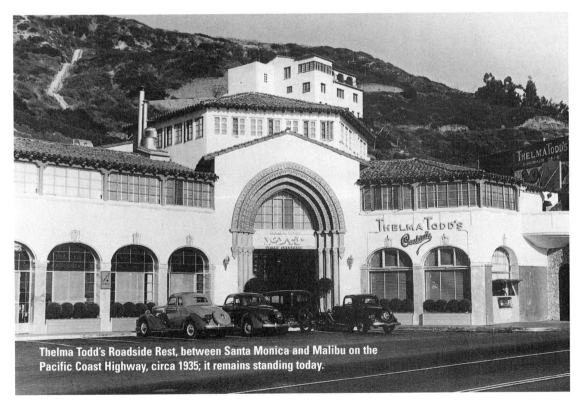

Thelma Todd's Roadside Rest, between Santa Monica and Malibu on the Pacific Coast Highway, circa 1935; it remains standing today.

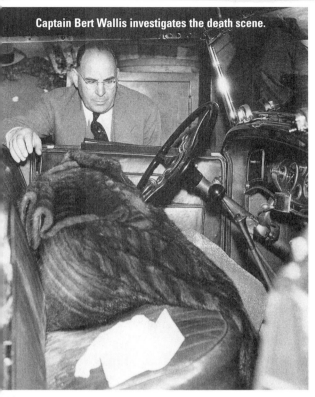

Captain Bert Wallis investigates the death scene.

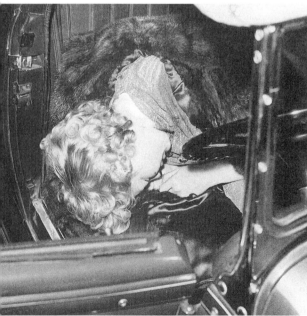

The coroner's inquest on Thelma Todd, more than 110 onionskin transcript pages in length, raises questions about both suicide and foul play, a definitive summary for one of Hollywood's greatest unsolved mysteries.

West's testimony in the inquest was shaky and, coupled with the ambiguity of their relationship, he became suspect. West told the coroner's jury that he slept in a separate room with a sliding door. He was asked, in a more civil and indirect 1935, if he was "an intimate friend" of Todd's and only admitted to being Todd's business partner. West had known her four years and put up the property and high-quality restaurant equipment to get the cafe going. Ironically, he'd bolted the one outside door that Todd had the key to for that night, which would have let her into the upper living area, above the cafe.

However, after driving Todd home after a party at approximately 3:15 in the morning, chauffeur Ernest Peters offered, as was his custom, to walk Todd up to her door from the Roosevelt Highway (now called Pacific Coast Highway) in Pacific Palisades. The normally cheery, talkative Todd had said nothing the entire trip and moodily replied, "No, never mind. Not tonight." It was at least 300 feet uphill and she never walked it alone. She was also subject to fainting spells.

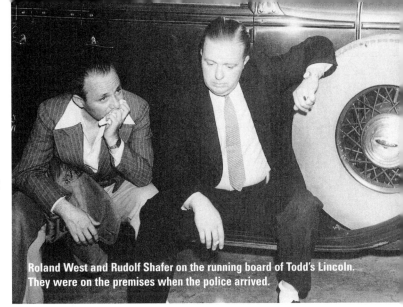

Roland West and Rudolf Shafer on the running board of Todd's Lincoln. They were on the premises when the police arrived.

Could Todd have committed suicide after being further disheartened by not getting into her own home? The keys were always left in the ignitions of both cars. But she had once before been locked out, and that time she'd broken a window and awakened a sleeping West.

Indeed, it had been a cold, windy night in the Palisades. Did Thelma Todd knock on the door, then march up to the garage, start the engine, perhaps to drive to her mother's, 10 minutes away in Santa Monica, and then fall asleep?

Bruce F. Clark, captain in the LAPD and first detective on the case, told the inquest questioners that there were no signs of struggle, no bruises on Todd's body. At the same time, there was no note, and no motive for suicide.

Rudolf Shafer, West's brother-in-law and manager of the cafe, reinforced the positivity of Todd's life at the time. He verified her joy for her recent Christmas shopping as well as her little-known plans to expand the upper floor to accommodate the booming business.

Related to these unfulfilled plans were the postmortem efforts of Todd's attorney. He believed the underworld was responsible and requested a second inquest. His theory was that mobster Lucky Luciano proposed that Todd convert her cafe into a secret gambling parlor; when she refused, he unleashed his vengeance. The inquest request was declined.

Could jealousy as a spurned/potential lover have been a motivational factor for West? Certainly, he contradicted himself in testimony. West insisted he heard running water in Todd's bathroom around 3:30 A.M. but did not find her in her room when he arose later in the morning. He then revised his statement and claimed Shafer told him the water noise "could have been the carbonator that pumps water to the fountain," downstairs in the cafe. Also unconvincing was West's initial assertion that his dog began whining just before the water sound and "never" whined as a habit. Some pages later, he changed his words, saying his dog whined every time its blanket came off.

A final, supernatural twist on this complex tragedy was the testimony of Todd's friend, Mrs. Wallace Ford. She claimed she'd received a call from Todd on Sunday afternoon, around 4:30. Todd had already been invited to a large party that had begun at 3:00 P.M. Todd, identifying herself on the phone by the nickname Ford had coined, "Hot Toddy," asked if she could bring a guest. Ford inquired if the guest was a girlfriend. The fun-loving Todd would not reveal any more than that the guest was male: "I want to have the fun of seeing your face when I come through the door."

But Todd never arrived because, according to the coroner's surgeon Wagner, she was dead sometime between four and five o'clock *that morning*. Even more curious, LAPD officer A. R. Kallmeyer, in the briefest appearance in the inquest, told those assembled that the phone records from Todd's home revealed no calls to Ford that day.

Recently but amicably divorced, Thelma Alice Todd Di Cicco was 29 years, 4 months, and 17 days old, when she died under the most mysterious of circumstances.

Bugsy Siegel

By the end of World War II, two notorious Coroner's Office cases had seared themselves into the fabric of L.A. lore, further embossed via books and films that have recently dealt

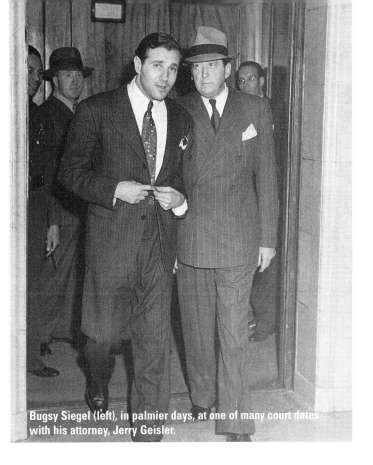

Bugsy Siegel (left), in palmier days, at one of many court dates with his attorney, Jerry Geisler.

with their bloody ends, *Bugsy* and *L.A. Confidential.*

A look at the two-page Coroner's Register number 37448 tells one that a Benjamin Siegel, 41, was found at 810 North Linden Drive in Beverly Hills. It further states that on June 20, 1947, at 10:50 P.M., Mr. Siegel's cause of death was "cerebral hemorrhage, due to gunshot wound of the head." There is no mention as to the victim's profession.

The New York gangster Benjamin "Bugsy" Siegel rode into town in 1936 and immediately miffed the studio brass. He coerced hundreds of extras (background actors) to pay him "union dues" and charged the studios whenever they drew from his pool of "organized labor." In one year, this illegal racket netted $500,000, which the mobster promptly invested in drug trafficking.

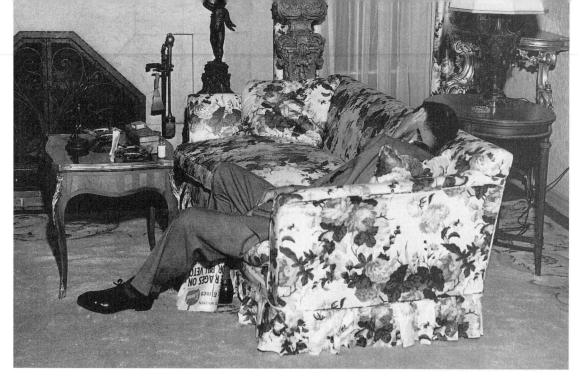

While gaining his nickname for a hair-trigger temper, no one who valued his well-being called him "Bugsy" to his face. In 1945, Bugsy persuaded a team of investors to pump $6

million into the construction of a hotel-casino out-side the sleepy desert town of Las Vegas. Two years later, the Flamingo blazed with gaudy neon grandeur, but none of the backers received a cent.

On that June evening in 1947, as Bugsy relaxed with a newspaper in his mistress's Beverly Hills home, machine-gun fire strafed the living room, drilling the gangster and the surroundings with lead. Although the mobster's murder remains unsolved, it has been confirmed that the gunmen were hired by infuriated Flamingo financiers.

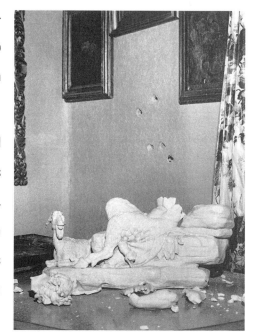

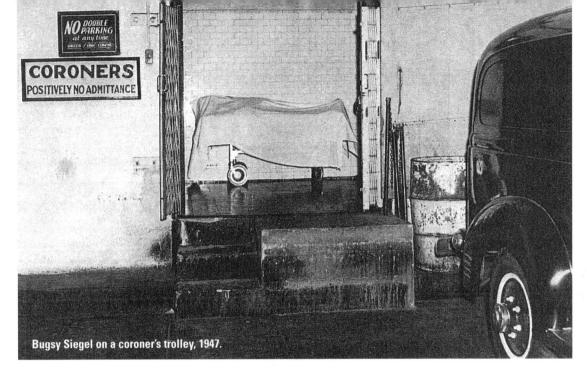

Bugsy Siegel on a coroner's trolley, 1947.

Listed as personal belongings received by the Coroner's Office:

"$408, billfold

W.M. wrist watch

Y.M. money clip

Y.M. chain, 6 keys & 1 room key

Y.M. ring with stone

W.M. cuff links (2)"

In listing an inventory of personal effects received, the Coroner's Office uses the abbreviations "W.M." for "white metal" or metal that is silver in appearance, and "Y.M." for "yellow metal," which may or may not be gold. Of course, no assumptions are made until effects are carefully examined, but in the case of the wildly wealthy and considerably greedy Bugsy Siegel, one could assume they were the real thing.

Elizabeth Short: "The Black Dahlia"

Six months before Bugsy Siegel was riddled with bullets, one of L.A.'s most infamous killings took place: the Black Dahlia Murder.

On January 15, 1947, near a weedy lot on the corner of 39th and Norton, at about 10:30 in the morning, as the sun was burning off the dew, a housewife was pushing her stroller

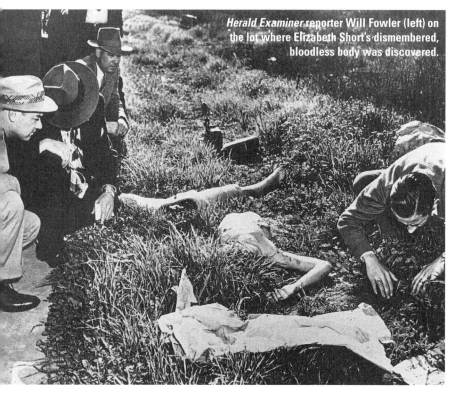

Herald Examiner reporter Will Fowler (left) on the lot where Elizabeth Short's dismembered, bloodless body was discovered.

past the shin-high grass. She spotted waxy, white limbs lying on the turf near the sidewalk. It looked like a mannequin, but on second glance, she realized it was the nude body of a young woman.

The victim had been cut in two and disemboweled, with the upper torso laying about 10 inches from the lower. The face was slashed with an ear-to-ear laceration, and the breasts bore gashes. There were also the telltale signs of torture: bruises, scratches, and rope burns on the neck, wrists, and ankles. But what truly horrified the patrolmen was the absence of blood.

By the time a Coroner's Office hearse pulled up and attendants put both halves of the victim into a conveyance casket, L.A. was growing alert to the news of its most horrific crime.

At the morgue, deputy coroners tagged the corpse Jane Doe Number 1, determined it weighed 115 pounds and was, in height, 5 feet, 5 inches. By late afternoon, fingerprints and a drawing of a formerly attractive young woman were sent to the press so they would appear in the next edition.

As L.A.'s largest circulation paper, the *Herald Examiner* wanted to break the story. At 4:00 A.M., the International News Photowire opened, and the *Examiner* used it to beam

photographs of the fingerprints to FBI headquarters in Washington, D.C. Within minutes, the Feds matched the prints with those found on a civilian job application filled out four years earlier at a Santa Barbara County army base. They wired back with the identity: Elizabeth Short, born July 29, 1924, in Hyde Park, Massachusetts.

At 10:40 that morning, the autopsy began. The surgeon determined the direct cause of death stemmed from massive hemorrhaging and shock. He

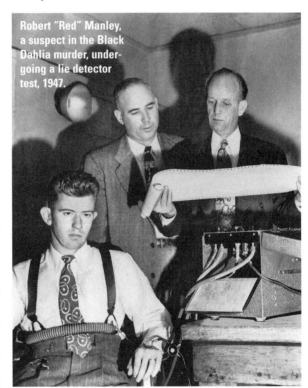

Robert "Red" Manley, a suspect in the Black Dahlia murder, undergoing a lie detector test, 1947.

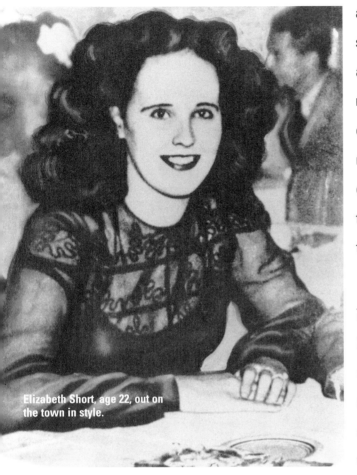

Elizabeth Short, age 22, out on the town in style.

also found more signs of torture. A piece of skin had been inserted into her vaginal canal, and her stomach contained digested fecal matter, suggesting she'd been forced to eat excrement while alive. But the question of rape went unresolved. The killer had thoroughly scrubbed the body, removing any traces of blood and semen, even shampooing the raven-black, shoulder-length curls.

Law enforcement responded *en masse*. Over 750 investigators from the LAPD, L.A. Sheriff's Department, and California Highway Patrol combed the county for the suspected torture chamber, scouring basements, attics, storm drains, and warehouses. Forty patrolmen canvassed the local neighborhoods, while 60 vice dicks raked downtown and Hollywood bars. A city councilman offered a $10,000 reward for information leading to the killer. Thousands of leads were investigated, over 150 known sex offenders were questioned, and the crime lab operated nonstop during the case's first week.

Detectives learned that a hardware salesman had driven Elizabeth Short from San Diego to Los Angeles on January 9 and dropped her off at the Biltmore Hotel, where she was last seen alive. The salesman, a 26-year-old with a wife and child, was promptly arrested, spent two days under intense interrogation, and collapsed from exhaustion during his second lie-detector test: He was found to be an innocent man.

The case had intrigued readers from the start with sensational headlines that screamed "Werewolf Murder" and "Vampire Killing." The *Herald Examiner* again scooped the competition by tracking down the Short family in Medford, Massachusetts. The reporter extracted information from Short's mother by saying her daughter had won a beauty contest and he needed background material for an article. When the reporter finally told the truth, Mrs. Short accused him of playing a cruel hoax, started to cry, and hung up.

The *Herald Examiner*'s city desk had the story, but now the editors, catching heat from publisher William Randolph Hearst himself, were clamoring for an accompanying photo. They sent a reporter skilled at cop impersonations to Santa Barbara, where he stumbled upon a mug shot of Elizabeth Short taken by Santa Barbara police four years earlier, when she had been arrested for underage drinking. Using the local paper's photowire, he sent it to the *Examiner* newsroom. Stunned, the editors gawked at the image of a drop-dead gorgeous brunette. She had a "haunting beauty," as one put it, one that abounded with newsstand appeal.

But the background story of Elizabeth Short didn't begin to unfold until after reporters learned she was called "the Black Dahlia" in L.A. club circles. It was discovered that the 22-year-old, who favored lacy, black clothing, theatrical hats, and heavy makeup, ran with a fast crowd, haunting Hollywood nightspots, sleeping until noon, and, on occasion, going to afternoon photo shoots. The movie *The Blue Dahlia* had just been released and, as a joke, friends tagged Short "the Black Dahlia."

With a year gone by and the crime still unsolved, the LAPD recklessly attempted to pin the murder on an innocent man. They even paraded him before a crowd of reporters, clapping on the cuffs as flashbulbs popped. The irate victim sued for $100,000; the grand jury launched an investigation that found the LAPD rife with corruption. The police chief was forced into retirement.

In the 1980s, a tipster approached the LAPD with information on a possible suspect, a man in his fifties or sixties, a downtrodden alcoholic who knew intimate details about the Black Dahlia murder. Days before an undercover meeting could be set up, the suspect was burned to death when a fire erupted in his skid row hotel room. Investigators believed the blaze ignited after the drunken suspect had passed out while smoking in bed.

The Lipstick Murder

As proof of the profound impact of the Black Dahlia murder, a similar case followed less than a month later. Dubbed the "Lipstick Murder," it featured another naked, mutilated female body, this time found in a field in West Los Angeles.

This second of what the press termed "werewolf killings" was nearly as vicious as Short's murder, for the victim had been kicked to death. Deep heel and sole impressions covered the face, chest, and hands, reducing the right side of the face to a pulp. The county autopsy surgeon revealed that one of several shattered ribs had pierced the heart.

For a final touch of desecration, the words FUCK YOU had been written in red lipstick

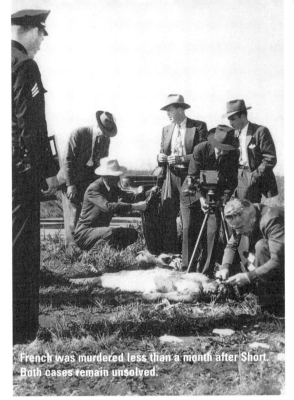

French was murdered less than a month after Short. Both cases remain unsolved.

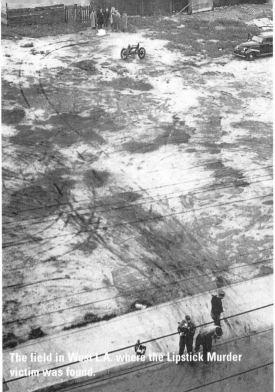

The field in West L.A. where the Lipstick Murder victim was found.

on the corpse's chest, with the letters BD scrawled just beneath, an obvious reference to the Black Dahlia and, possibly, a copycat killer.

Unlike the aimless, young Elizabeth Short, this victim turned out to be a minor celebrity. Jeanne Axford French, 40, had been a onetime actress and, later, a pioneering aviatrix. Her recent life had consisted of an unhappy marriage to one Frank French, who worked at an aircraft plant in Culver City. Both were heavy drinkers and fought with each other constantly. Mr. French, however, was questioned and soon cleared as a suspect in the murder.

A coroner's jury ruled the death of Jeanne French, like that of Elizabeth Short, to be "homicide by a person or persons unknown." These two most odious murder cases in Southern California's history remain officially open, as does the lingering question of whether they could have been committed by the same person.

Sam Rummel: "The Great Mouthpiece"

During the '30s and '40s, when a corrupt City Hall and paid-off policemen worked hand-in-glove with organized crime, Sam Rummel was the attorney of choice for many a mobster and cop on the take. After World War II, Rummel achieved true celebrity status as the close friend and busy advocate of L.A.'s star gangster, gambling czar Mickey Cohen. Rummel himself was part owner of several casinos in Reno and in Gardena. "The Mob's Mouthpiece" thrived on the company of his dangerous clients, but ultimately this perverse infatuation led to his death.

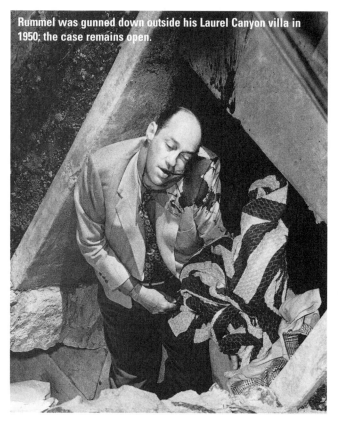

Rummel was gunned down outside his Laurel Canyon villa in 1950; the case remains open.

By 1950, the U.S. government's investigations into organized crime had set their sights on Los Angeles. One of their main targets was a finance company that was the front for a huge bookmaking operation run by Cohen associates, advised by Rummel. The "company" worked out of a storefront on East Florence Avenue in county territory.

Investigators seized the finance company's ledgers, which revealed a $108,000 payoff to police and

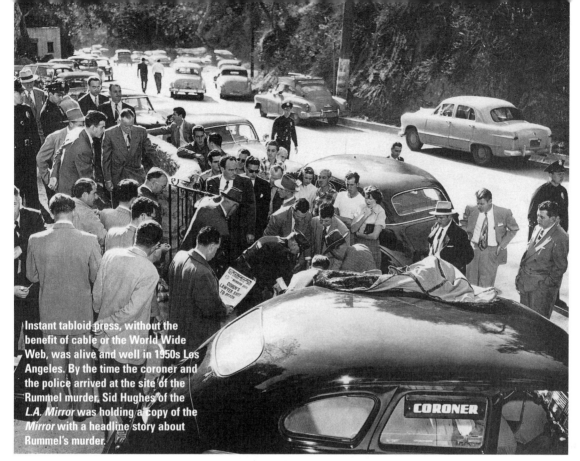

Instant tabloid press, without the benefit of cable or the World Wide Web, was alive and well in 1950s Los Angeles. By the time the coroner and the police arrived at the site of the Rummel murder, Sid Hughes of the *L.A. Mirror* was holding a copy of the *Mirror* with a headline story about Rummel's murder.

sheriffs. Suspicion fell on a vice squad captain, as well as a sheriff's captain who more than once had ordered deputies in the vice squad (which was not his department) to "lay off" the bookies. Both were called as witnesses; both stammered and came off looking guilty as hell. One "retired" soon thereafter; the other was yanked off the vice squad.

By early December, Sam Rummel knew that an L.A. grand jury investigation was imminent. On December 11, the very worried "retired" captain summoned Rummel for a secret meeting with himself and two others from the sheriff's office.

What was said can only be surmised; what happened afterward may have been the result of that meeting.

Rummel arrived home late that night, pulling into the driveway of his "lavish villa" (as

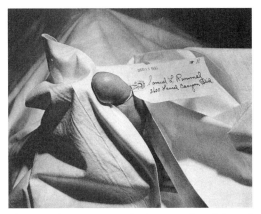

the papers called it) on Laurel Canyon Boulevard at about 1:30 A.M. As he walked to the front door, a loud blast rang out. Rummel died on the walkway by an iron gate; six shotgun pellets were in his neck. The spread of the blast was 14 inches in diameter. The coroner's official cause of death is recorded as "hemorrhage, due to gunshot wounds of head and neck, inflicted by a shotgun in the hands of some person or persons at present unknown."

The weapon was found early the next morning across the street, lodged in the crook of a tree, apparently used by the assailant to steady his aim. As for the assailant, he was never found and the murder of Samuel L. Rummel remains unsolved.

Someone, with a lot to lose, had silenced the "Great Mouthpiece."

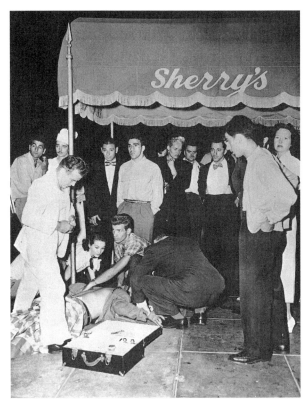

Rummel's client, gambling czar Mickey Cohen, was also a target. Outside of the Sunset Strip nightclub Sherry's, Cohen's aide, Eddie "Needle" Herbert, was shot in the back; Cohen and bodyguard Harry Cooper were wounded.

Johnny Stompanato

Like the previous decade, the 1950s closed with the flowing of infamous blood. Actress Lana Turner had one of her greatest performances in the 1942 film *Johnny Eager*, in which she was the love interest to a suave but ruthless gangster, played by Robert Taylor. Life imitated art, as Turner's dalliance with mobster Johnny Stompanato turned into a series of threats of violence.

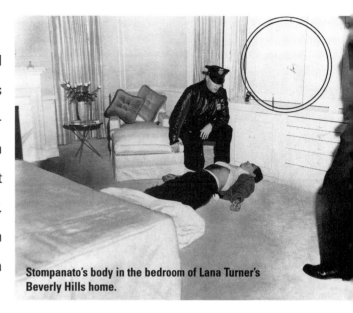

Stompanato's body in the bedroom of Lana Turner's Beverly Hills home.

With sharp Latin features and Italian charm, Stompanato was nicknamed "Johnny Valentine" by his underworld friends. He'd been Turner's boyfriend for about a year, but their relationship had been increasingly rocky.

According to Coroner's Office files, a call from Turner's mother came in at 11:25 P.M. on April 4, 1958. Investigators rushed to Turner's Beverly Hills home at 730 North Bedford Drive to find the lifeless figure of Stompanato in the second-floor bedroom.

Stompanato lay on his back, his arms outstretched in the middle of the bedroom. A stab wound in his abdomen had penetrated his aorta and liver. While there was little blood near the body, investigators discovered in the bathroom sink a bloody, 10-inch kitchen knife. In a bedroom, they came upon Turner's 14-year-old daughter, Cheryl Crane, whimpering, "I didn't mean to kill him." No one believed the gangly adolescent could have stabbed to death the hardened gangster.

Physically, Cheryl was 5 feet, 8½ inches tall and weighed between 130 and 135 pounds. She had an athletic build and, at the time, had been wearing bra, slip, and bathrobe and watching television.

Stompanato was 32 years of age, six feet tall, weighing 176 pounds. His olive complexion was set off with black hair and brown eyes. The coroner's report noted his dress, which was typical for the flashy gangster: He wore an orange-rust sweater (Springle of Scotland from Simpson Piccadilly) and under it, a gray shirt with silk collar (Monte Factor Ltd. of Beverly Hills), where one could find a bloodstain and 1¼-inch cut in the stomach region. He wore black socks (Genuine Palm Beach label) and handmade shoes from a London shop (Bespoke shoes), which, oddly, featured cleats on the bottom. The supine figure also had a bloodstained lady's white handkerchief on him, as well as a white hand

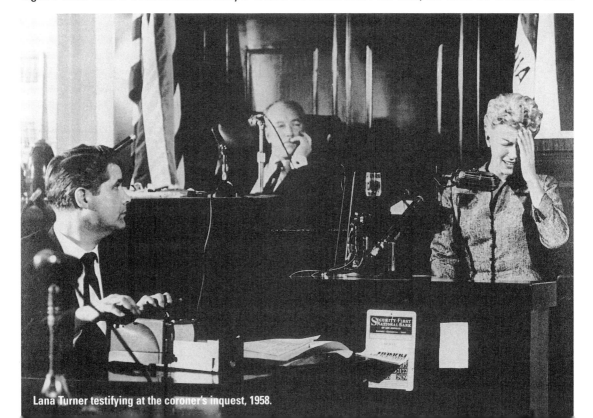

Lana Turner testifying at the coroner's inquest, 1958.

towel (Cannon terry cloth), used by Turner to staunch the flow of blood.

But this description could not reveal what Turner herself portrayed, the actual sequence of events, in great detail, in her testimony at the coroner's inquest.

At the coroner's inquest, Evelyn Marcocchio reenacts the murder of Stompanato with attorney William Jerome Pollack looking on.

Between 2:00 and 4:30 P.M. that day, Stompanato had taken Turner shopping in Beverly Hills. Friends later joined Turner at her home, where Stompanato remained until 5:45. Turner's daughter, Cheryl, who was on Easter break from Happy Valley School in rural Ojai, had been with her father Steven Crane, and returned to Bedford Drive at 5:30. Turner's friends left between 7:00 and 7:30 P.M.

Stompanato called at 7:50 to say he "was coming over."

When he arrived after eight, Stompanato was angry about the amount of time Turner had spent with her friends. Turner testified she went to her daughter's room to avoid his "saying some very bad things." When asked if he was threatening her at that point, she replied, "Well, no, the threat wasn't there but the language was bad."

Stompanato's tirade continued, prompting Turner to say, "Not in front of the baby," referring to the teenage Cheryl. The lovers went downstairs and Turner pleaded for him to leave. He would not and they returned to the upstairs, where Turner, out of patience, insisted, "I can't go on like this. No more. Leave me alone."

Enraged at the idea of being dumped, Stompanato grabbed Turner by the arms and shook her and cursed, making threats of violence against her and her daughter. Turner then noticed Cheryl in the doorway. "Please, Cheryl. Please don't listen."

"Are you sure, mother?" came the concerned reply.

Turner repeated the request and closed her bedroom door. From behind the door came more shouting, including Turner's pronouncement, "Don't ever touch me again! I'm absolutely finished! Get out!"

It was at this point Turner claimed she opened the bedroom door to send Stompanato on his way, and Cheryl suddenly appeared, running past her mother.

"I thought she hit him in the stomach," Turner testified.

Stompanato grabbed his abdomen at the wound, turned one-half position, and dropped onto his back. Turner got the towel from the bathroom and put it over the wound, hearing gurgling in the victim's throat. Turner then called her mother and asked her to call their family doctor, Dr. McDonald.

Cheryl was sobbing, "Mama, I didn't mean to do it." She left her mother's room and went to call her father. Turner slapped Stompanato's face lightly, to try and revive him, but the gurgling continued.

Crane arrived first and took Cheryl from the horrific bedroom scene. Turner's mother came next, but left before police arrived. When Dr. McDonald showed up at Bedford Drive, he called an associate named Dr. Webber. Two attendants also came. Adrenaline was administered to Stompanato—too late. McDonald asked Turner to call attorney Jerry Geisler, a social friend of Turner's. Then, after all this mayhem, Police Chief Anderson of Beverly Hills was notified.

The coroner's testimony regarding the body cited 1,500 cc's of clotted blood and fluid in the peritoneal cavity. The wound was $5\frac{1}{2}$ inches deep, from the skin to termination against the vertebral column. Stompanato had been in normal health, although, curiously, his kidneys were four times the normal size.

Further inquest and file documents provide a fuller picture of the event and its seeming inevitability. Malevolent rumors circulated after Stompanato's death, suggesting that Turner murdered him and arranged for Cheryl, a minor, to take the rap. Eric Root, in his book *The Private Diary of My Life With Lana*, claims Turner herself told him it was the truth. It is a known fact that when the police arrived at Bedford Drive, Turner, hysterical, was tearfully begging, "Can I take the blame?"

Cheryl was quoted by police as saying, "I stabbed him. Didn't mean to kill him. Just frighten him."

Turner admitted there had been many previous verbal fights in front of Cheryl, including one on the day before the incident.

Turner had ironically just moved into Bedford Drive, after a trip overseas. Earlier in London, it was learned at the inquest, Stompanato had threatened Turner with a razor.

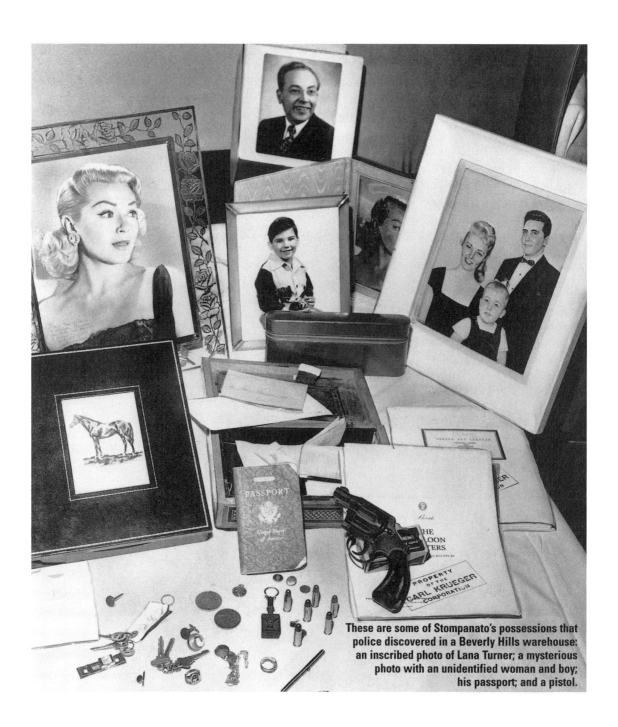

These are some of Stompanato's possessions that police discovered in a Beverly Hills warehouse: an inscribed photo of Lana Turner; a mysterious photo with an unidentified woman and boy; his passport; and a pistol.

Cheryl was appalled upon hearing this and felt that the relationship was making her mother ill.

In a final twist of fate, the knife, which possessed a smudged fingerprint, was never purchased. The house had come furnished, with the 10-inch knife in its kitchen.

The coroner's jury ruled it a justifiable homicide—committed by Cheryl Crane.

George Reeves

Actor George Reeves became famous for his television portrayal of comic strip hero Superman. But, far from being the Man of Steel in his private life, Reeves shot himself in the head under strange circumstances on June 16, 1959.

Born George Keefer Brewer, Reeves was adopted by his stepfather and took the name George Bessolo until he landed his first major role in the film classic *Gone With the Wind*.

At about midnight on June 16, Reeves prepared to go to sleep at his home at 1579 Benedict Canyon. His houseguests, Robert Condon and Leonora Lemmon, were left to retire to their separate bedrooms. This alone was suspect, as Lemmon was Reeves's fiancée and she claimed they were to be married on Friday of that week. Yet, here was a showbiz figure, having her sleep in a separate room.

At about 12:05, Reeves's friend Carol Van Ronkel arrived with a William Bliss, admitted by Miss Lemmon. According to testimony, Reeves came downstairs in a bathrobe, angered by the late, unexpected arrival. Bliss apologized to Reeves, who in turn apologized for his own outburst.

Here is where the LAPD Death Report, found in the Coroner's Office file, creates a great deal of suspicion. Lemmon's statement included this: "…As he (Reeves) went up the stairs, I said, 'In a moment, you will hear a gun. See, there, the dresser drawer is opening and he is getting the gun out. Now you will hear the shot.' Just then, I heard the gun fire and Mr. Bliss went upstairs to see how Mr. Reeves was."

The obvious questions not asked of Lemmon were:

1) How did you know Reeves was going to shoot himself?

2) How could you hear what he was doing upstairs behind a closed door?

It is pertinent to examine the difference in Bliss's verbatim statement: "He [Reeves] had gone upstairs and had closed the door, when Miss Lemmon said, 'He is probably going to shoot himself.' I heard a drawer opening and she said, 'See, there he is, opening the drawer to get the gun.'"

Van Ronkel's statement is even more disconnected:

"…Mr. Bliss and I came down to the house to have a drink. There was some arguments and I don't know where everyone was when he went upstairs. I was not in the room."

Now, the LAPD report adds even more mystery:

"At this time, husband of witness [Van Ronkel] arrived and sent her home. Officers were unable to get any further statement from her at this time."

Again, there was an obvious, unasked question: If Van Ronkel is married, what is her relationship to Mr. Bliss, with whom she's unexpectedly visiting Reeves at midnight?

Reeves's Report of Chemical Analysis revealed .27 percent ethanol in his blood, but there were no notes or statements as to why he'd put a .30 German luger to his right temple and pull the trigger. Condon told police, "He was despondent due to lack of work, but I did not think he was despondent to the point he would shoot himself."

Further complicating the story was Reeves's longtime affair with Toni Mannix, wife of MGM executive Eddie Mannix. Hopefully, some light will be shed on the demise of the 45-year-old who could not compete with his heroic, television alter ego. The file has been officially reopened.

Marilyn Monroe

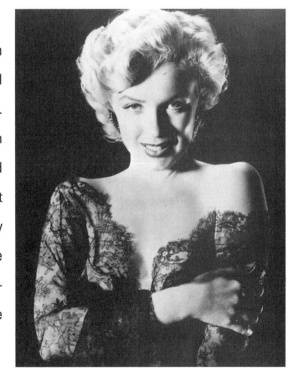

A string of unnerving deaths rocked L.A. in the 1960s, exacting a psychological toll equal to any of the city's shattering earthquakes. On August 5, 1962, screen siren Marilyn Monroe was found dead in her Brentwood home. To this day, her affairs with President John F. Kennedy and his brother, Attorney General Robert F. Kennedy, as well as some contradictory forensic evidence, have promulgated the theory that her official suicide may have unofficially been murder.

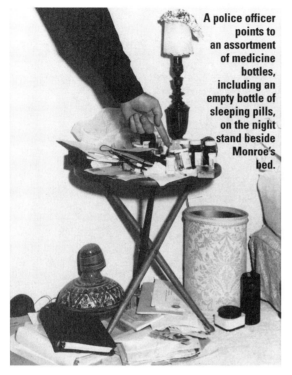

A police officer points to an assortment of medicine bottles, including an empty bottle of sleeping pills, on the night stand beside Monroe's bed.

Coroner's Case #81128 looked on the surface to be open and shut. The 36-year-old actress had, in her blood, according to the toxicological study, 4.5 mg percent barbiturates and 8.0 mg percent chloral hydrate. In her liver, pentobarbital registered at a level of 13.0 mg percent.

Coroner Theodore Curphey released a statement on August 17, which includes a summary report by a psychiatric investigation team of three doctors, Robert Litman, Norman Farberow, and Norman Tabachnick. In part, it reads, "In our investigation, we have learned that Miss Monroe had often expressed wishes to give up, to withdraw, and even to die. On more than one occasion in the past, when disappointed and depressed, she had made a suicide attempt using sedative drugs. On these occasions, she had called for help and been rescued."

The strongest forensic doubt cast upon the autopsy conclusion of "acute barbiturate poisoning, ingestion of overdose" may be the question of why no barbiturate was found in Monroe's stomach, despite the blood and liver levels and the empty bottle of Nembutal next to her.

Robert Slatzer, writer and longtime friend of Monroe's, has written a letter in the file, addressed to L.A. County supervisor Mike Antonovich, who initiated an investigation into Monroe's death in 1981. This 1985 letter from Slatzer summarizes some major inconsistencies.

For one, Walter Schaefer, owner of the Schaefer Ambulance Company, insisted they received a call at 2:00 A.M. to pick up Monroe at her home at 12305 Fifth Helena Drive, where she was delivered to Santa Monica Hospital, died in emergency, and then inex-

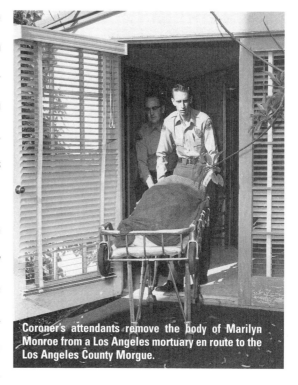

Coroner's attendants remove the body of Marilyn Monroe from a Los Angeles mortuary en route to the Los Angeles County Morgue.

plicably wound up back at the house, naked, prone on the bed, with a telephone in her hand. Without explaining this, housekeeper Eunice Murray has corroborated the ambulance picked up Monroe and her body arrived back at the house before the police were called.

Also of note is the testimony of Deborah Gould, former wife of Monroe's friend Peter Lawford. She insists Lawford and an investigator went to Monroe's house to "clean things up" and that Lawford destroyed a note she had written. Gould also states Lawford told her, "Marilyn took her last big enema." Monroe had been taking enemas to facilitate bowel movements, but this reference was interpreted by Gould as regarding an enema of Nembutal, which could have accounted for the lack of barbiturate in her stomach.

Antonovich prompted District Attorney John Van de Kamp's 1982 review of the case, which reads, in part, "The facts, as we have found them, do not support a finding of foul play."

This review was motivated by former Coroner's employee Lionel Grandison, who claimed that he was coerced into signing Monroe's death certificate, that the investigation was incomplete, and that a red diary he saw at the Monroe residence disappeared from the Coroner's Office two days later.

But a December 1982 report in Coroner's Office files, from Assistant District Attorney Ronald Carroll and Investigator Alan Tomich, refutes Grandison's claims: "Mr. Grandison was discharged from the Coroner's Office a short time after the Monroe autopsy for misconduct involving the theft of property from dead bodies." Grandison pled guilty to one count of forgery.

The report also asserts, "The story of the red diary first publicly appeared in Slatzer's book (*The Life and Curious Death of Marilyn Monroe*). Slatzer claimed to have seen it and to have discussed with Miss Monroe the contents of her diary, including references to Robert Kennedy, Fidel Castro, the CIA, etc. Excluding Mr. Grandison's belated statements concerning the diary, Slatzer is the only source alleging the existence of the document."

The possibility of a lethal injection or "hot shot" can be ruled out, as Dr. Thomas Noguchi examined Monroe's body with a magnifying glass eight hours after the discovery of the corpse and found no needle marks. In the Carroll–Tomich report, John Miner, then deputy district attorney, claims he was present with Noguchi. Miner interviewed Monroe's psychiatrist, Dr. Ralph Greenson. The 1982 Carroll–Tomich report says, "In essence, Greenson believed that Miss Monroe appeared to be making progress, on a psychiatric level, and Greenson said that she had been making plans for the future...whatever the circumstances, an intentional overdose did not fit with her psychological profile."

One indisputable fact is that Monroe's status as a vulnerable, sexual icon is made all the more potent by the questionable details of her sudden, sad departure.

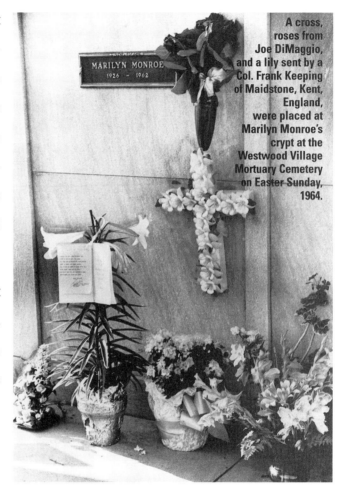

A cross, roses from Joe DiMaggio, and a lily sent by a Col. Frank Keeping of Maidstone, Kent, England, were placed at Marilyn Monroe's crypt at the Westwood Village Mortuary Cemetery on Easter Sunday, 1964.

Dorothy Dandridge

Hailed as more than just a black sex symbol, Dorothy Dandridge was a triple threat—dancer, singer, actress. Her lofty perch as the first African-American woman to be nominated for an Academy Award descended tragically to a death that tested the forensic capabilities of the Los Angeles County Coroner's Office. Found in her Sunset Strip residence at 8495 Fountain Avenue, apartment D2, on September 8, 1965, the light-skinned Dandridge had on nothing but a blue scarf.

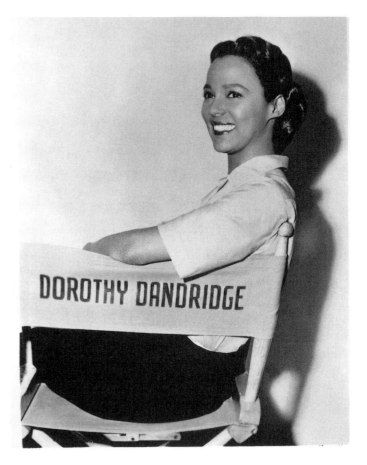

Highlighting her career was an Oscar nod in the 1954 all-black musical *Carmen Jones*. Dandridge was originally dragged into Hollywood and showbiz by her mother, Ruby, who decided to leave her Cleveland marriage and, accompanied by a domineering lesbian lover, make stars of Dandridge and her sister Vivian.

It was originally concluded that Dandridge had died as a result of a toe fracture that released bone marrow into her bloodstream. As a September 10, 1965, press release from Charles Langhauser, senior inquest deputy at the Coroner's Office stated: "Final cause of death has been determined as due to a fractured right metatarsal with pulmonary and cerebral fat emboli as the result of an accidental fall, fracturing a bone in the right foot."

Dandridge's manager, Erwin Mills, confirmed in a sheriff's department report in the files that she had slipped on some stairs on September 3 at Terry Hunt's Gym, which prompted her foot being taped and her using crutches. Mills called her on the fateful day twice in the morning, but Dandridge skipped having a cast put on, claiming she was very tired and needed to sleep. Calling numerous times in the late afternoon, Mills eventually used a crowbar to open the chained door and find Dandridge face down on the bathroom floor, a wet washcloth near her face.

The coroner's conclusion might have stood, if not for the questioning reactions of forensic associates, including letters in the files from Dr. William Sturner, associate medical examiner of New York, and Dr. Alfred Angrist from Albert Einstein College of Medicine, Yeshiva University in the Bronx.

Reconsidering the possibility of the embolism from that extremity, Coroner Theodore Curphey utilized the Armed Forces Institute of Pathology (AFIP) in Washington, D.C., whose toxicological report found the newly marketed antidepression drug Tofranil in Dandridge's tissue and blood. But there was not a sufficient amount to cause death. Brigadier General Joe Blumberg, the AFIP's director, also stated in his November 15 report, "...no fat emboli in lung or brain." He went on to declare "...there is no satisfactory explanation for the demise of this individual." Curphey's press release of November 17 announced the official cause as "Acute Drug Intoxification" due to Tofranil.

If it was drug-induced, was it suicide or accidental? Dandridge had not been in a major film since *Porgy and Bess* in 1959, and, despite having worked as a performer for 39 of her 42 years, she was bankrupt.

Yet, she had just gone to Mexico with Mills to discuss doing two pictures in that country. Dandridge had seemed in good spirits and had been quite active since a leukemia scare in May.

The final mystery regarding Dorothy Dandridge relates back to that blue scarf. The Coroner's Office file on Dandridge features a curious, yellowing *L.A. Herald Examiner* story in the files, dated October 11. Manager Mills told of being given, on May 21, a quickly scrawled will, which read: "In case of my death to whomever discovers it—don't remove anything I have on—scarf, gown, or other [crossed out] underwear. Cremate me right away. If I have anything money furniture give to my mother Ruby Dandridge. She will know what to do."

Hauntingly, Mills said she handed the sealed envelope to him and told him, "You keep it, Earl, because I know you will be the one who discovers me." Mills insisted in a police report that this will was due to Dandridge being rattled by the then-recent death of friend Nat King Cole and her own leukemia scare. A hematologist had in fact put Dandridge's worries to rest shortly thereafter; medical science, however, cannot know what was in the star's mind as she pressed that wet washcloth to her face.

Robert Kennedy

Near midnight on June 5, 1968, Senator Robert F. Kennedy walked through a crowd of cheering supporters in the Ambassador Hotel ballroom at 3400 Wilshire Boulevard, having won the California Democratic primary election. It was seemingly assured that Kennedy would follow his slain brother's role as president of the United States.

But as he entered the pantry, he was hit by three bullets, apparently fired from a .22 caliber revolver by Sirhan Bishara Sirhan. Struck twice in the torso and once in the head,

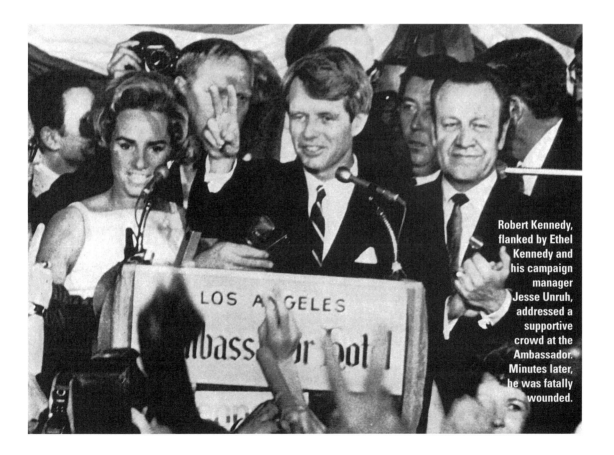

Robert Kennedy, flanked by Ethel Kennedy and his campaign manager Jesse Unruh, addressed a supportive crowd at the Ambassador. Minutes later, he was fatally wounded.

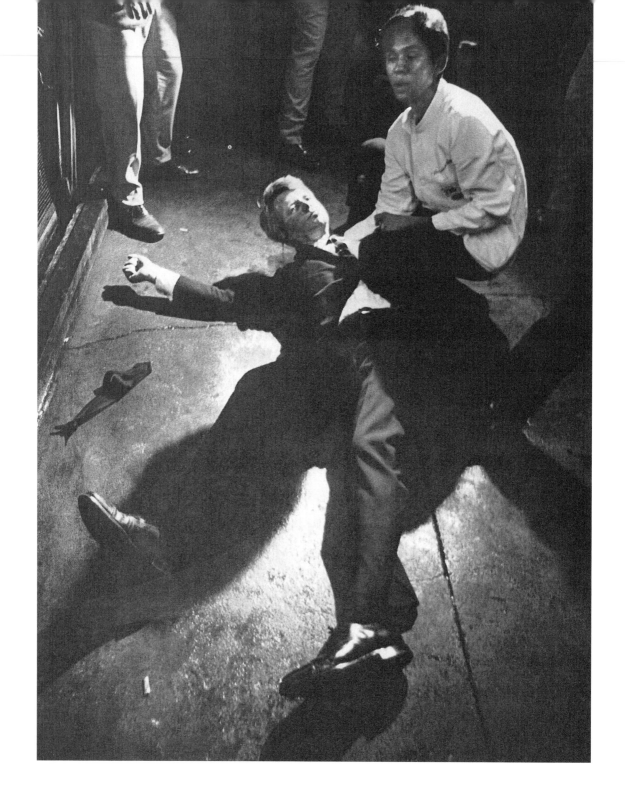

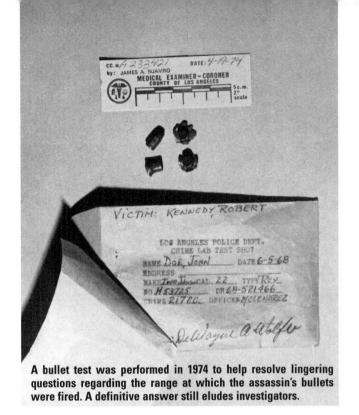

A bullet test was performed in 1974 to help resolve lingering questions regarding the range at which the assassin's bullets were fired. A definitive answer still eludes investigators.

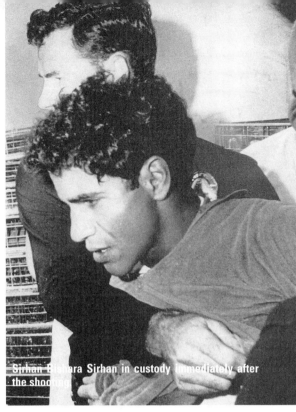

Sirhan Bishara Sirhan in custody immediately after the shooting.

the 42-year-old Democratic Party hopeful died at 3:00 A.M., June 6, at Good Samaritan Hospital. According to the autopsy report signed by Thomas Noguchi, death was ascribed to "gunshot wound of right mastoid, penetrating brain."

An hour before Kennedy succumbed, the coroner had secured the hospital to prevent Secret Service men from spiriting the corpse away to Washington, as they did after John F. Kennedy's assassination in Dallas.

At the autopsy, performed at 3:00 A.M., minutes after the Senator's demise, the coroner followed the deadly bullet's trail into the brain. It had pierced the skull near the right ear, leaving a scattering of microscopic, metallic fragments. These were immediately collected and stored. The autopsy was praised for its thoroughness, which is evident when reading the 62-page document.

Yet, as with his brother's murder, Robert Kennedy's has much controversy surrounding it. Among the many questionable facts is the removal of wall panels in the Ambassador's pantry before a full investigation could be performed and the disappearance of armed Wackenhut security guard Thane Cesar, who was in close proximity to Kennedy at the time of the shooting.

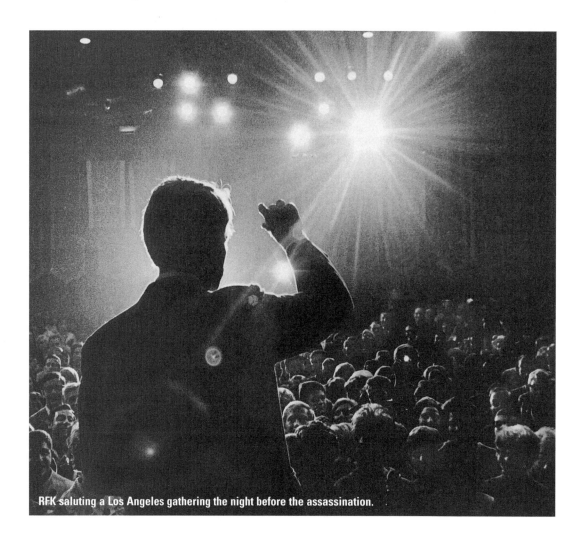

RFK saluting a Los Angeles gathering the night before the assassination.

Sharon Tate

The turbulence of the 1960s was capped off with a group of killers whose grisly acts permeate the American conscience to this day. Just after midnight on August 9, 1969, four members of the "Manson family," the cult headed by messianic figure Charles Manson, broke into the Bel Air estate of Sharon Tate, the 26-year-old film actress and pregnant wife of director Roman Polanski. Wielding knives and pistols, the intruders killed Tate and her four friends in a stunningly savage fashion.

The Manson murders came at a time of total upheaval in American society. Twenty days before, U.S. astronauts had taken their first hopeful steps on the moon, yet violence besmirched the globe. In 1969, the first draft lottery was instituted, as the number of U.S. military dead in Vietnam approached 40,000. Unarmed Black Panther Fred Hampton was killed by Chicago police under questionable circumstances. Sirhan Sirhan and James Earl Ray faced sentencing in connection with the murders of Robert F. Kennedy and Martin Luther King. Thirty-one Soviet troops were killed in a border clash with China that was threatening to escalate. Even in the world of music, events were spiraling out of control: The

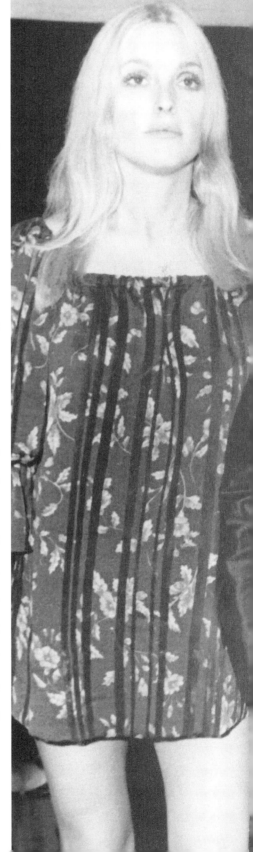

Rolling Stones concert at California's Altamont Speedway was marred by the murder of a man at the hands of the Hell's Angels. Mick Jagger had been beaten by a member of the motorcycle gang.

The butchery at 10050 Cielo Drive in Bel Air, as administered by the Svengali-like Manson and his LSD-influenced minions, is made all too vivid when consulting both coroner's photos and autopsy reports. Tate, about to give birth to a boy in one month, had 16 stab wounds across her

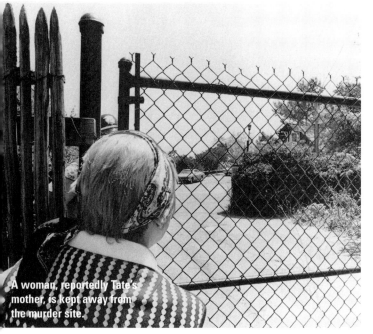

A woman, reportedly Tate's mother, is kept away from the murder site.

chest, back, abdomen, both arms, and right thigh. A nylon cord around her neck was looped over a beam of an upstairs sleeping loft. The cord was also tied around the neck of hair stylist Jay Sebring.

Also included in the file is a transcript of Thomas Noguchi's trial testimony, as questioned by prosecutor Vincent Bugliosi. Regarding the condition of Tate's face, Noguchi stated: "Abrasions are around the left cheekbone and following the curvature of the cheekbone back to the ear..." It was concluded she had been hung by the rope for a time after her murder.

Noguchi ordered the rope to be cut to facilitate moving Tate and Sebring. The latter had seven stab wounds to his chest and back, and facial contusions. Via X rays, a bullet was found in Sebring's chest, with fragments of it near his spine. The Coroner's Medical Report cited the same knife being used on Tate and Sebring; it was found in front of the living room fireplace on blood-soaked carpeting, with broken effects throughout the room.

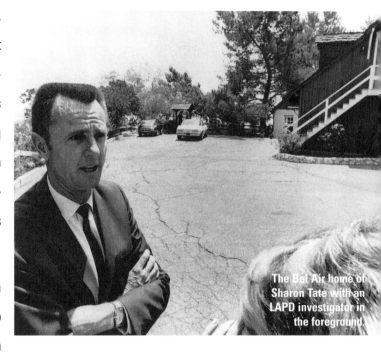

The Bel Air home of Sharon Tate with an LAPD investigator in the foreground.

The Coroner's Medical Report gave a sense of the other victims' attempts to flee. Heiress Abigail Folger was found on the lawn outside, on her back, wearing only a white dressing gown. Her autopsy report contained 21 documented stab wounds, as well as seven others discovered later. The Preliminary Examination Report noted fly eggs in the hair at the back of her head and the Final Autopsy Report attributed her death to a stab wound to the aorta, causing exsanguination (death by loss of blood). The Report of Chemical Analysis revealed that Folger was under the influence of drugs at the time, with a reading of 2.4 percent mg of methylene dioxy amphetamine (MDA), a psychedelic. Folger, who had done social work for her last job, would have been 26 two days later, on August 11.

No more than 60 feet from Folger lay Polish writer Voityk Frykowski, in front of the veranda on the lawn. Clearly the most maimed, his body eventually yielded under scrutiny

51 separate stab wounds, a gunshot wound to the back, a later-documented shot in the left leg, and 13 head lacerations. Like Folger, Frykowski's Report of Chemical Analysis revealed MDA (though a lesser amount of 0.6 percent mg) by a test of his urine. The back gunshot

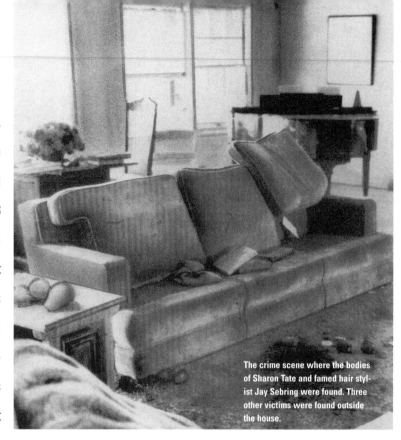

The crime scene where the bodies of Sharon Tate and famed hair stylist Jay Sebring were found. Three other victims were found outside the house.

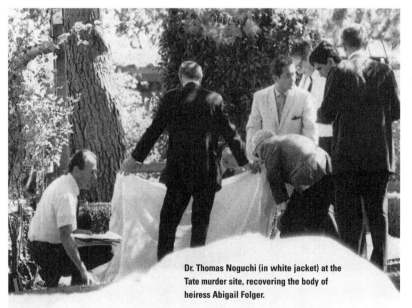

Dr. Thomas Noguchi (in white jacket) at the Tate murder site, recovering the body of heiress Abigail Folger.

alone was fatal, let alone the seven stab wounds to both of his lungs.

Steven Earl Parent was the youngest of the Cielo Drive victims. According to the Coroner's Medical Report, the 18-year-old, redheaded clerk made it all the way to the driver's seat of his late model Rambler Ambassador, parked at the entrance gate. The anatomical survey section of the autopsy report found two fatal gunshot wounds, causing perforation of his left lung, trachea, aorta, and thorax. A third, nonfatal bullet entered the left side of his face, and there was an incised knife wound on his left hand. The inventory of Parent's personal effects revealed a pen, class ring, glasses, and 90 cents in change.

Leaving behind five brutalized bodies, no weapons, and the word PIG spelled in blood on the front door, the Manson "family" had imprinted an ugly, indelible mark on the country's imagination. But it did not end there.

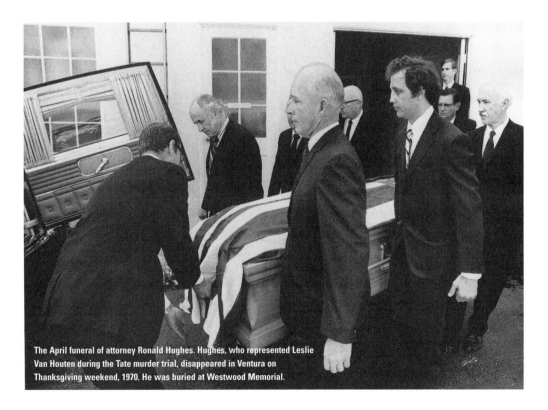

The April funeral of attorney Ronald Hughes. Hughes, who represented Leslie Van Houten during the Tate murder trial, disappeared in Ventura on Thanksgiving weekend, 1970. He was buried at Westwood Memorial.

Leno and Rosemary La Bianca

The very next day, August 10, the "family's" carnage continued in the Los Feliz (Spanish for "the happy") section of Los Angeles. At 3301 Waverly Drive, a winding, secluded street, the bodies of Leno and Rosemary La Bianca, dressed for bed, were found at 10:20 P.M. by their son, daughter, and the daughter's fiancé.

The Coroner's Medical Report on the La Bianca killings is based on information from Officer Galindo of the LAPD, who was at the scene. Leno, owner of the Gateway chain of supermarkets, was lying on the floor between two couches, a two-pronged fork from a carving set stuck superficially into his abdomen. The word WAR had been crudely carved into his lower chest and his head was wrapped in a white, bloody pillowcase, secured by an electrical cord still attached to a large table lamp.

On the front wall, near the upper left corner of the door, the word RISE was spelled in blood, as was the phrase DEATH TO PIGS, on the back of the living room wall. Recalling a wild, intense Beatles song and leading to a

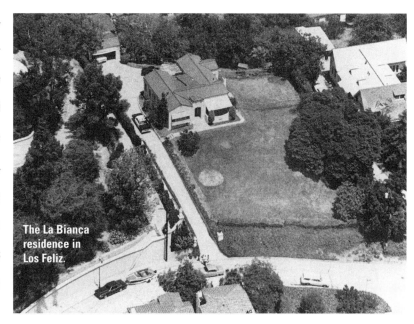

The La Bianca residence in Los Feliz.

title for Bugliosi's book on the cases, the misspelled HEALTER SKELTER was written in blood on the La Bianca refrigerator.

Mrs. La Bianca was found in the bedroom, also with her head covered in a pillowcase, tied with a lamp cord. The police differ as to whether she wore a nightgown or pajama top, but it was described as raised above her buttocks, revealing a series of stab wounds and scratches. The lamp and lamp table were askew, with some dollar bills and other effects scattered on the bedroom floor.

Officially, the autopsy report attributed the 44-year-old Leno La Bianca's death to "multiple stab wounds to neck and abdomen." This time, a weapon was left. The knife had a wooden handle $4\frac{1}{2}$ inches long and a blade $4\frac{7}{8}$ inches long, serrated on one edge. It had been used to stab him 13 times. The fork had created seven pairs of double tine wounds. There was also a ligature around one wrist.

Rosemary La Bianca, 38, had the following listed on her autopsy report: 22 upper back stab wounds, 14 wounds on her lower back, 4 on her anterior trunk, and 1 on her lower right mandible (jaw).

Stray hairs were obtained from Mrs. La Bianca's hand. Yet, what helped break the case, ironically, was information supplied in jail by accomplice Susan Atkins, told in confidence to a cell mate. During the trial, it was established that Manson was not present at the Tate site but did witness the La Biancas being tied up. He then walked outside and told his followers to "kill them." All the Manson defendants received death sentences, but later had them commuted to life imprisonment when California's laws were changed.

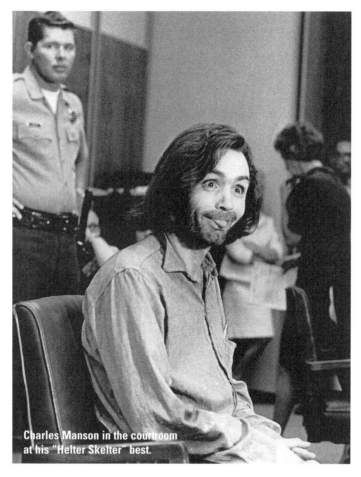
Charles Manson in the courtroom at his "Helter Skelter" best.

The macabre nature of the killings will remain a gory Southern California legacy with the permanence of the X's purposely carved into the foreheads of Manson and his bewitched followers. If any of these cult members are ever to be paroled, the most likely candidates are Atkins, an accomplice, not a murderer, and Leslie Van Houten, whose stab wounds to Mrs. La Bianca were performed after La Bianca's death, presumably at the urging of the other members of her "family."

Ruben Salazar

The years 1969 and 1970 were so filled with violent demonstrations and bombings that they were dubbed, by certain radical activists, as "The Days of Rage." It was an appropriate name for the events in predominantly Latino East Los Angeles on August 29, 1970, as a

Chicano protest against the war in Vietnam led to a riot and the death of *Los Angeles Times* columnist and Spanish language television station KMEX news director Ruben Salazar.

Salazar was covering the Chicano Moratorium Committee's antiwar protest in Laguna Park. According to Hunter S. Thompson's coverage in *Rolling Stone* and his book, *The Great Shark Hunt*, the rally was peaceful until a handful of Chicanos engaged in fights with the police, bringing a one-hour fusillade of rocks, bottles, bricks, and other items thrown at the cops. Then, the police exploded, with tear gas, batons, and even 12-gauge shotguns. The crowd fled and torched and looted the main thoroughfare, Whittier Boulevard.

Salazar and his on-camera associate Guillermo Restrepo were in the Silver Dollar Bar at 4945 Whittier, preparing their story, when 50-year-old Manuel Lopez directed a sheriff's deputy, Thomas Wilson, to the bar, claiming he saw two men with guns enter the bar. Wilson ordered the patrons to leave the bar with a bullhorn, but no one heard inside.

Wilson waited 5 or 10 minutes, then fired Flite Rite tear gas projectiles through the black curtain in the doorway of the Silver Dollar. One glanced off the doorway but the other two entered the darkened interior. Salazar had just ordered a beer from a stool near the entrance, while Restrepo used the men's room. According to the autopsy report, he died of "projectile wound to left side of head causing skull fracture and extensive cerebral destruction." Half of Salazar's head was blown away from the impact.

The community would be further incited, as the sheriff's office would at first claim Salazar died of sniper and/or "errant gunfire" in Laguna Park. It was also learned that after the patrons of the bar had run out the back, Salazar's body remained in the bar for hours before, at a local resident's urging, deputies found the murdered journalist. Additionally that day, Gilbert Diaz, 30, had died of a gunshot wound after trying to run a barricade. Lynn Ward, 15, was killed by an explosive device in a trash bin that was so powerful, it hurled him across Whittier Boulevard through a plate glass window.

There was a coroner's inquest into the death of Salazar and it created as much drama for its time as the Simpson–Goldman trial would in the '90s. Seven VHF and two UHF stations carried the televised coverage in shifts. Hearing Officer Norman Pittluck twice refused to sign a subpoena to obtain the sheriff's office manual on use of tear gas weapons, which Salazar attorney Douglas Dalton called "really absurd."

From the first of 15 total days, emotions ran high. A new group of jurors had to be impaneled when an overanxious press started asking the original jurors questions the minute they sat down. A blue-ribbon committee of 21 Mexican-Americans walked out that first day, calling the inquest "a sham," after extensive sheriff's office testimony. Throughout, many did not understand that in an inquest, because rules of evidence do not apply, hearsay and rumor were included.

A Mexican Independence Day march went ahead on September 16. With Salazar's name being invoked, the parade of 2,500 in front of a crowd of 200,000 nearly made it to the end. But violence again broke out. At least 72 were injured, including 33 deputies.

After 61 witnesses, 204 exhibits, and 2,025 pages of testimony, the October 8, 1970, *L.A. Times* reported four jurors voting Salazar's death "at the hands of another person." Three voted "accident." All jurors admitted to being unsure. District Attorney Evelle Younger refused to prosecute or in any way discipline Deputy Wilson.

Despite the tragedy, the East L.A. Hispanic community became politically galvanized. Ruben Salazar, who served as war correspondent in Vietnam and the Dominican Republic, now has a library that bears his name in the barrio of East L.A.

Janis Joplin

Considered the greatest white blues singer of her time, Janis Joplin had fused blues, rock 'n' roll, and folk into a powerful mixture that culminated in her San Francisco band Big Brother and the Holding Company hitting number one on the charts in November 1968 with the album *Cheap Thrills*.

Significantly, too, the Top 20 hit on the album was titled "Piece of My Heart," for it was the performer's sensitivity that led to her drug-induced demise in Hollywood on October 4, 1970, in a hotel with the cruelly ironic name "The Landmark."

Joplin had left college in Austin, Texas, with a great deal of resentment, after a fraternity had viciously named the then-overweight, acne-ridden singer "Ugliest Man on Campus." Janis not only developed her hard-drinking, wild-living alter ego "Pearl" over the next two years of travel, she also obtained a rather intense reliance on methamphetamine or "speed." Joplin did return to her hometown of Port Arthur for a brief while, due to alcohol and drugs getting the better of her during her first stay in the Bay Area. But, by the time the "San Francisco Sound" had culturally blossomed and Big Brother had their breakthrough at the Monterey Pop Music Festival in 1967, she had found a belated acceptance for her bohemian dress, highly emotional singing, and wildly sexual stage energy.

But Joplin, tired of "shucking and jiving" and making less money than she deserved, left, with great difficulty, the protective womb of Big Brother. She first formed the Kozmic Blues Band and then the Full Tilt Boogie Band, releasing records with both. By 1970, she was dependent upon not only her signature Southern Comfort bottle but the use of heroin.

Working on her album *Pearl* in Hollywood, Joplin often frequented the rock hangout Barney's Beanery on Santa Monica Boulevard in West Hollywood. After finishing a session after midnight on October 4, she headed to Barney's and had two drinks. According to the manager at the Landmark, Joplin was in good spirits as she arrived at 7047 Franklin Avenue around 1:00 A.M. and headed up to apartment 105. When the manager noticed her car was still in its stall at seven that evening, he called Joplin's apartment. Getting no answer, he let himself in and found her on the floor next to the bed.

Dr. Thomas Noguchi was one of the three scene investigators. Discovered was a rubber glove in a basket with white powder, dried blood on gauze, and a disposable towel.

In another area of the room was a hypodermic kit with a teaspoon with a black smudge on it, along with cotton with dried residue on it. Also found: a needle with plastic syringe containing clear liquid. In a dresser drawer in the living room was a paper packet of brownish-white powder. The Joplin site also had a bag of marijuana and a bag with four and a half small white tablets.

The official coroner's report listed Joplin's death as "acute heroin, morphine overdose and intoxication."

Many have speculated as to whether the death of Joplin, like other rock stars, was intentional or accidental. Her sometimes raucous exterior belied an inner vulnerability, one that, despite sexual relationships with both men and women, once prompted her to say, "Onstage, I make love to 25,000 people. Then I go home alone."

In her biography *Buried Alive*, author Myra Friedman cites Joplin asking a onetime, Bay Area boyfriend Seth Morgan, whom she once considered marrying, to help her get off heroin.

Further enhancing the mystery of Joplin's death is the fact that three days before, on October 1, 1970, she had executed a new will, with specific instructions about an eventual cremation.

Janis Joplin died at the age of 27.

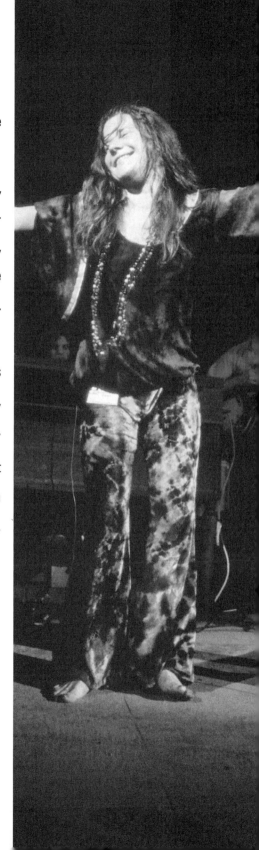

Donald DeFreeze—a.k.a. "Cinque"

Events leading up to L.A.'s deadliest gunfight started February 4, 1974, when members of the terrorist group the Symbionese Liberation Army, led by escaped convict Donald DeFreeze, kidnapped 20-year-old publishing heiress Patricia Hearst from her Berkeley apartment. In lieu of ransom, the SLA demanded that her father, newspaper magnate William Randolph Hearst Jr., donate over $400 million to the poor, a demand Hearst wouldn't meet.

Negotiations between the SLA and Hearst continued for two months, but then, in a strange twist of events, Patricia announced she had joined her captors to fight for the freedom of all oppressed people. Days later, she and seven comrades robbed a San Francisco bank.

Months later, Los Angeles police were tipped off that the group had hunkered down in a South Central L.A. bungalow, and on May 17, about 500 flak-jacketed law officers surrounded the hideout. A furious gunfight erupted, with waves of automatic rifle fire spraying the area for

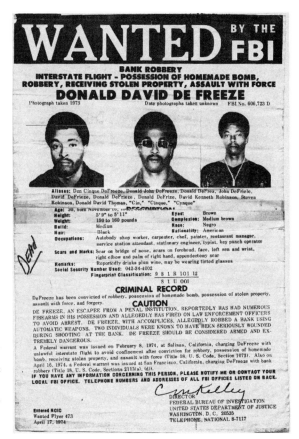

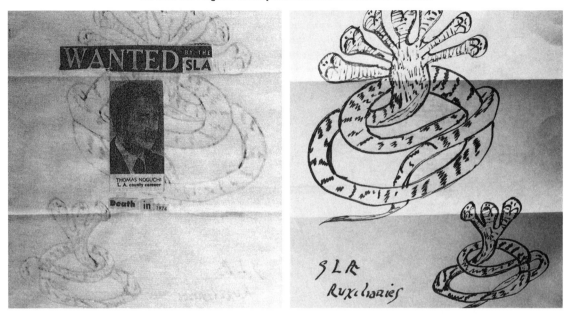

two hours until the little house burst into flames, charring the six inhabitants beyond recognition.

With the fire extinguished, the coroner's team raked the ashes for the victims' remains, while Hearst and his friend, then-Governor Ronald Reagan, urged the coroner to learn if Patricia had been in the flame-engulfed structure. Since fingerprints no longer existed, the forensic team obtained the dental records of all suspected SLA members and compared them to the teeth recovered from the embers. Within two days, the team identified each victim. DeFreeze had used the name "Cinque" after an African slave who led a revolt against his white captors. Originally identified by the Coroner's Office as "John Doe #4," DeFreeze's positive identification required his dental cards from the Southern Reception Center at Chino, California's prison. Patricia Hearst would be caught at a later date in San Francisco.

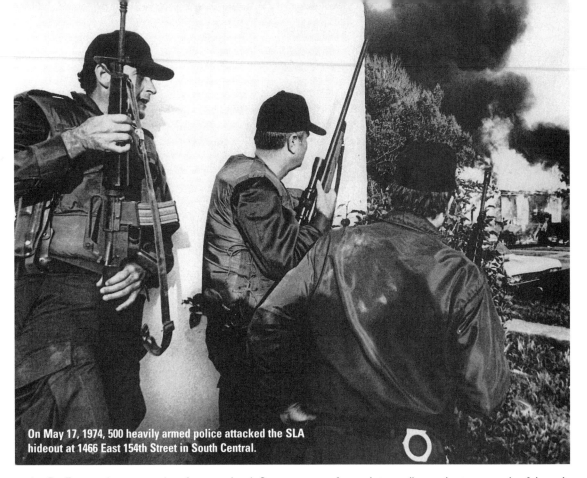

On May 17, 1974, 500 heavily armed police attacked the SLA hideout at 1466 East 154th Street in South Central.

In DeFreeze's case, the Anatomical Summary referred to a "gunshot wound of head, through brain, fatal." This was in addition to serious burns and wounds from exploding ammunition. DeFreeze was dressed for war. The autopsy report described in part "…a heavy canvas ammunition pouch, a large metal and plastic bayonet sheath and a black compass in a canvas casing. Behind the ammunition pouch, there is attached a 4" long, broken hacksaw blade."

But one vexing question remained. Did DeFreeze meet his end from a police bullet or his own? The coroner's team applied an electron microscope to glean trace metals from the death-inflicting bullet hole. In a report from the Forensic Science Center, while the conclusion did not categorically credit the police, the following phrase does lead to an answer: "Note that in the decedent's GSW [gunshot wound] we found little evidence of primer residue. This observation...suggests that the lethal bullet was not discharged at contact distance."

Often overlooked in discussion of the SLA and Hearst was the shady motivation of DeFreeze. He had been an informant for the Criminal Conspiracy Section (CCS) of the LAPD. Furthermore, the book *The Phoenix Program* by Douglas Valentino details mind control techniques used at Vacaville Medical Facility, allegedly in order to program black

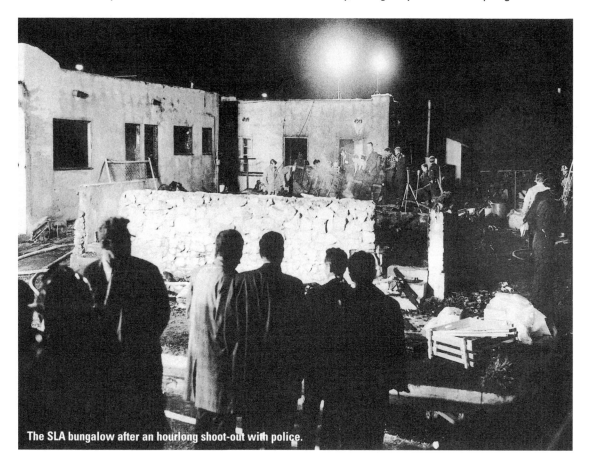

The SLA bungalow after an hourlong shoot-out with police.

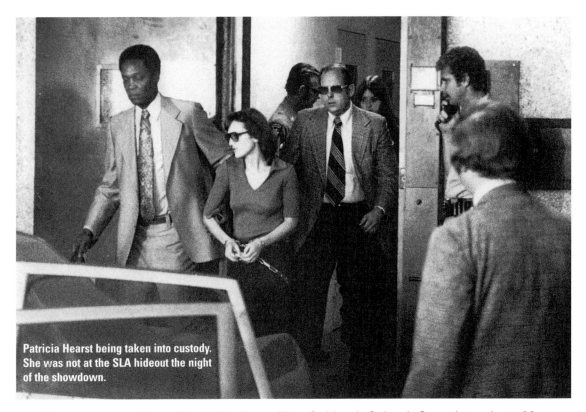

Patricia Hearst being taken into custody. She was not at the SLA hideout the night of the showdown.

convicts to assassinate black leaders, like Oakland School Superintendent Marcus Foster and Black Panthers Bobby Seale and Huey Newton. DeFreeze himself once claimed to be under the influence of drugs and mind control on Vacaville's top-secret third floor. Head of the front organization the Black Cultural Association, he was transferred inexplicably to a different prison, where he broke out the very next day and immediately formed the SLA.

Freddie Prinze

One of the rare cases in which a civil court jury voted for a different conclusion than the Coroner's Office came after the January 28, 1977, death of television star Freddie Prinze. Despite the wealth and fame that his series *Chico and the Man* had brought him, the comedian was found at a mere 22 years of age with a self-inflicted bullet wound to the right temple, while his business manager was present at 3:30 A.M. in Prinze's apartment 216 at his 10300 Wilshire Boulevard residence in West Los Angeles.

There is no doubt Prinze had been depressed. His pending divorce from his wife, Kathy, as well as his concerns about his career had driven Prinze to threaten suicide before. When Marvin "Dusty" Snyder, his manager, received a call at 2:45 A.M. from Prinze saying, "I'm going to end it all," Snyder's measured reply was that they had a meeting at 10:30 that morning. Prinze then insisted, "You won't see me there." This prompted Snyder to come to Prinze's apartment at three in the morning.

Snyder observed the troubled television star toying with a loaded .38 Astra automatic. They talked briefly and Prinze made several phone calls, the last to Mrs. Prinze, who testified to the LAPD he said, "This is it, honey."

Mrs. Prinze responded, "Don't talk like that."

"I mean it this time," he stated and hung up the phone and pulled the trigger.

The Coroner's Case Report verifies Prinze had been loading and unloading the gun in front of secretary Carol Novak and spoke briefly that day with his psychologist.

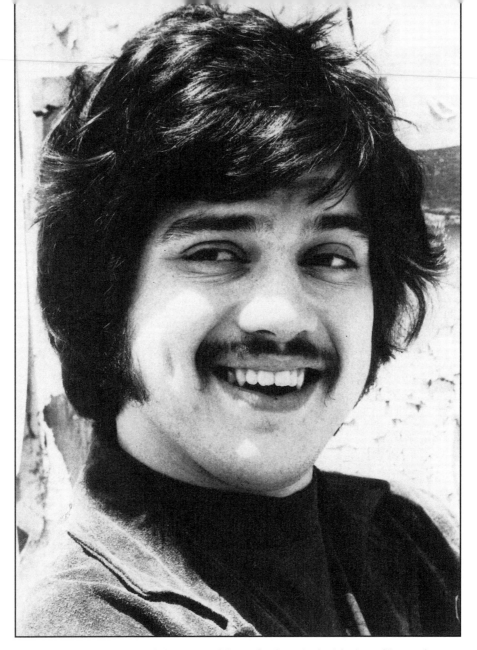

Prinze was found sitting straight up on his sofa, hands in his lap. Not only was a spent projectile found four feet from him, but another was on the floor near the bathroom door-jamb. This bullet, apparently fired in distraction or by accident earlier, was lodged in a dresser in the dining room.

The controversy regarding Prinze surrounded his Report of Toxicological Analysis, which revealed .42 mg percent of methaqualone (quaaludes) in his liver. Further, the Medical Report mentioned IV punctures on both arms, though no other drugs were found in blood or tissue.

Prinze also left a suicide note, in a shaky handwriting, which read, "I must end it. There's no hope left. I'll be at peace. No one had anything to do this [sic]. My dicision totaly [sic]. Freddie Prinze. P.S. I'm sorry. Forgive me. Dusty's here. He's innocent, he cared."

A civil court took the level of drugs and desperate, scrawled handwriting as an indication of Prinze not being in control of his own actions, ruling the death "accidental."

But in a February 4, 1983, letter in the files to Prinze attorney Martin Friedlander, who asked for an official cause change from suicide to accident, Dr. Joseph Choi, assistant acting chief of the Forensic Medicine Division, on behalf of Acting Coroner Dr. Ronald Kornblum, refused to do so. The letter cites Prinze's "history of depression over his marital problems, the report of police investigation, the autopsy findings, the report of psychological autopsy and, most of all, the clearly stated suicide note."

A sad addendum to the Prinze file is a newspaper clipping, dated February 3, 1977, from the *Van Nuys Valley News and Green Sheet*. Lynn Barillier, 13, of La Crescenta, distraught over idol Freddie Prinze's death, left a note to that effect, prior to picking up her father's .38 pistol and ending her own life.

Karen Carpenter

With an angelic, pure vocal gift and, along with her brother Richard, a group that was one of the best-selling musical acts in America between 1970 and 1980, Karen Carpenter seemed to have the life dreams were made of. They sold over 100 million units and toured internationally throughout the '70s. And yet, Karen Carpenter battled anorexia nervosa for a year and a half. Oddly, she had seemingly con-quered the illness, gaining weight and looking healthy, when she collapsed and died in the Los Angeles suburb of Downey on February 4, 1983.

The Coroner's Case Report lists that Karen Anne Carpenter was 32 years of age when she was found, unresponsive, on the floor of her walk-in bedroom closet in her parents' home at 9828 Newville, and that she died at Downey Community Hospital.

The Interdepartmental Work Sheet in her file listed her newest doctor as George

CERTIFICATION OF VITAL RECORD

COUNTY OF LOS ANGELES • REGISTRAR-RECORDER/COUNTY CLERK

CERTIFICATE OF DEATH
STATE OF CALIFORNIA

0190-012181

LOCAL REGISTRATION DISTRICT AND CERTIFICATE NUMBER

1A. NAME OF DECEDENT—FIRST	1B. MIDDLE	1C. LAST	2A. DATE OF DEATH	2B. HOUR
Karen	Anne	Carpenter	FEBRUARY 4, 1983	0951

3. SEX	4. RACE	5. ETHNICITY	6. DATE OF BIRTH	7. AGE
Female	White	American	March 2, 1950	32

8. BIRTHPLACE OF DECEDENT	9. NAME AND BIRTHPLACE OF FATHER		10. BIRTH NAME AND BIRTHPLACE OF MOTHER
Connecticut	Harold B. Carpenter	China	Agnes R. Tatum Maryland

11. CITIZEN OF WHAT COUNTRY	12. SOCIAL SECURITY NUMBER	13. MARITAL STATUS	14. NAME OF SURVIVING SPOUSE
U.S.A.	564-82-9174	Married	Thomas J. Burris

15. PRIMARY OCCUPATION	16. NUMBER OF YEARS	17. EMPLOYER	18. KIND OF INDUSTRY OR BUSINESS
Recording Artist	12	Self - employed	Music

USUAL RESIDENCE

19A. USUAL RESIDENCE—STREET ADDRESS	19B.		19C. CITY OR TOWN
2222 Avenue of The Stars			Los Angeles

19D.	19E. STATE	20. NAME AND ADDRESS OF INFORMANT
Los Angeles	California	Richard L. Carpenter - Brother

PLACE OF DEATH

8341 Lubec Street
Downey, California 90240

AMENDED 1 of 2

21A. PLACE OF DEATH	21B. COUNTY
DOWNEY COMMUNITY HOSPITAL	LOS ANGELES

21C. STREET ADDRESS	21D. CITY OR TOWN
11500 BROOKSHIRE	DOWNEY

CAUSE OF DEATH

22. DEATH WAS CAUSED BY: (ENTER ONLY ONE CAUSE PER LINE FOR A, B, AND C)		24. WAS DEATH REPORTED TO CORONER
IMMEDIATE CAUSE (A) DEFERRED		83-1611
CONDITIONS, IF ANY, WHICH GAVE RISE TO THE IMMEDIATE CAUSE, STATING THE UNDERLYING CAUSE LAST. DUE TO, OR AS A CONSEQUENCE OF (B)		25. WAS BIOPSY PERFORMED? NO
DUE TO, OR AS A CONSEQUENCE OF (C)		26. WAS AUTOPSY PERFORMED? YES

23. OTHER CONDITIONS CONTRIBUTING BUT NOT RELATED TO THE IMMEDIATE CAUSE OF DEATH	27. WAS OPERATION PERFORMED FOR ANY CONDITION IN ITEMS 22 OR 23? TYPE OF OPERATION DATE
	NO

PHYSICIAN'S CERTIFICATION

28A. I CERTIFY THAT DEATH OCCURRED AT THE HOUR, DATE AND PLACE STATED FROM THE CAUSES STATED. I ATTENDED DECEDENT SINCE / LAST SAW DECEDENT ALIVE	28B. PHYSICIAN—SIGNATURE AND DEGREE OR TITLE	28C. DATE SIGNED	28D. PHYSICIAN'S LICENSE NUMBER
28E. TYPE PHYSICIAN'S NAME AND ADDRESS			

INJURY INFORMATION

29. SPECIFY - ACCIDENT, SUICIDE, ETC.	30. PLACE OF INJURY	31. INJURY AT WORK	32A. DATE OF INJURY	32B. HOUR

33. LOCATION	34. DESCRIBE HOW INJURY OCCURRED

CORONER'S USE ONLY

35A. I CERTIFY THAT DEATH OCCURRED AT THE HOUR, DATE AND PLACE STATED FROM THE CAUSES STATED, AS REQUIRED BY LAW I HAVE HELD AN INVESTIGATION.	35B. CORONER—SIGNATURE AND DEGREE OR TITLE	35C. DATE SIGNED
	S. Forman DEPUTY CORONER	2-5-83

36. DISPOSITION	37. DATE—MONTH, DAY, YEAR	38. NAME AND ADDRESS OF CEMETERY OR CREMATORY	39. EMBALMER'S LICENSE NUMBER AND SIGNATURE
Entombment	Feb 8, 1983	Forest Lawn, Cypress 4471 Lincoln Ave., Cypress, California	Ed Wilking 6985

40. NAME OF FUNERAL DIRECTOR	41. LOCAL REGISTRAR—SIGNATURE	42. DATE ACCEPTED BY LOCAL REGISTRAR
Forest-McKinley Downey 9830 Lakewood Blvd. #1081		FEB 9 1983

STATE REGISTRAR

VS-11 (10-78) 9315

01-9-4-3743

This is to certify that this document is a true copy of the official record filed with the Registrar-Recorder/County Clerk.

Charles Weissburd
CHARLES WEISSBURD
Registrar-Recorder/County Clerk

FEB 26 1993
19-1090840

This copy not valid unless prepared on engraved border displaying the Seal and Signature of the Registrar-Recorder/County Clerk.

Monnet, who had her on Ativan (2 mg) and the diuretic Lasix. Monnet had previously prescribed Quaalude and Demerol to Carpenter. He had last seen her January 10 and she had appeared in good health.

Karen ironically had begun to recover from her anorexia nervosa, an affliction most common in over-achieving young women between 18 and 25. Her Case Report listed her as weighing 108 pounds, which was a marked improvement for her.

Ironically, Karen had been plump as a child. A natural tomboy who loved sports, Karen hated gym class at Downey High and Richard helped her take band instead, where she marched in the drum line with a glockenspiel and eventually asked her parents for a drum set. She took choir to avoid geometry.

When Herb Alpert at A&M Records heard The Carpenters demo tape in April 1969, he signed them; their first significant hit, "Close to You," went to number one in six weeks.

The Coroner's Office had questioned Monnet about Karen's death: "Doctor suspects that patient may have been taking Lasix and not taking her potassium and therefore may

National Medical Services, Inc.
P.O. Box 433A, 2300 Stratford Ave.
Willow Grove, Pennsylvania 19090
(215) 657-4900

March 23, 1983

Dr. Ernest Griesemer
Department of Chief Medical Examiner-Coroner
1104 N. Mission Road
Los Angeles, CA 90033

Dear Doctor Griesemer,

On 2/16/83 we received from your Department, via Federal Express, one sealed and labelled container of blood and one of liver from your autopsy #83-1611.

In accordance with your request and on the basis of the history furnished us by you, that this was a possible delayed anorexia nervosa death, we analyzed samples from these two specimens, specifically for the constituents which you indicated, and obtained the results shown below in tabulated form.

A. Findings:

	Blood	Liver
Emetine	Negative (detection limit: 0.05 micrograms/g)	0.48 micrograms/g
Lorazepam (Ativan^R)	0.020 micrograms/mL	Not measured
Sulfisoxazole (Gantrisin^R)	6 micrograms/mL	Not measured
Furosemide (Lasix^R)	Negative (detection limit: 0.01 micrograms/mL)	Not determined
Tetracycline (Component of Mysteclin-F^R)	Negative (detection limit: 0.5 micrograms/mL)	Not determined
Doxycycline (Vibra-Tabs^R)	Negative	Not determined

B. Methods of Analysis:

Emetine: Screening of the blood by fluorescence spectrophotometry and high performance thin layer chromatography. Detection and measurement in the liver by high pressure liquid chromatography.

Lorazepam: Gas chromatography on 3 different columns with flame ionization and nitrogen selective detection.

Sulfisoxazole: Spectrophotometry.

Furosemide: Fluorescence spectrophotometry and high pressure liquid chroma-
                 tography with ultraviolet absorbance detection.

Tetracycline: Fluorescence spectrophotometry.

Doxycycline: Fluorescence spectrophotometry.

C. Comments:

1. Emetine is the major alkaloidal constituent of ipecac. It is used
    medicinally as amebicide. As a constituent of ipecac, it is
    an emetic, acting as such at a dose of 10 to 20 mg (e.g. in 15
    mL syrup of Ipecac). Emetine is potentially toxic to all tissues
    upon prolonged (even therapeutic) use, particularly uncoupling
    of phosphorylation in skeletal and cardiac muscle, thereby producing
    damage to subcellular organelles which can result in polyfocal necrosis,
    i.e., in the case of the heart, in toxic myocarditis. (Pathology
    of Drug-induced and Toxic Diseases, R.H. Riddel, ed., Churchill
    Livingstone, 1982.)

    In the course of chronic use of ipecac or emetine, the latter
    accumulates in the liver. Detectable concentrations in urine
    have been noted as much as two months after the drug has been
    discontinued. In a case of chronic ipecac syrup for 3 months
    which resulted in death following a period of hospitalization, 1.1
    micrograms emetine/g liver have been reported. (J. Amer. Med. Assoc.
    243: 1927, 1980).

    Thus in the present case, the finding of 0.5 micrograms emetine/g
    liver, with none detected in the blood, is consistent with
    residua of the drug after relatively remote cessation of its chronic
    use.

2. Lorazepam is used as a psychosedative in daily doses of 1 to 10 mg, which
    produce steady state concentrations between 0.1 and 0.3 micrograms/mL
    blood. It has a half life of around 12 hours.

    The concentrations of lorazepam (0.02 micrograms/mL blood is
    congruent either with a residue from remote chronic use of the drug
    or a peak blood level which occurs approximately 2 hours after a
    single 2 mg dose.

3. Sulfisoxazole, when used as an anti infective is maintained at a blood level of 50
    to 100 micrograms/mL.

    In the present case, the concentration of 6 micrograms/mL blood, is
    essentially at the low end of the reporting limit and thus, is
    consistent with remote use of sulfisoxizole.

4. Furosemide, is a diuretic with an onset of action within an hour after usual
    oral dosage of 20 to 40 mg (in renal failure up to 250 mg) and a
    duration of diuretic action of 4 to 6 hours after each dose. Diuresis
    is accompanied by potassium-- and calcium loss (as well as of other
    electrolytes). Thus, it can result in general fluid and electrolyte im-
    balance after either large single doses or prolonged administration.

---

have had a cardiac arrythmia." On the Certificate of Death, however, the phrase "Emetine cardiotoxicity" appears. A laboratory in Pennsylvania had tested both blood and liver for the Coroner's Office and found in the latter .48 mg/g emetine, "the major alkaloidal constituent of ipecac." Carpenter had used ipecac syrup to induce vomiting per her anorexia for so long, that even though she'd stopped, the fibers of her heart were pale and thin with large nuclei. "Thus, in the present case," summarized the lab results, "the finding of 0.5 micrograms emetine/g liver, with none detected in the blood, is consistent with residua of the drug after relatively remote cessation of its chronic use."

The only question that remained was a more personal one—why the multiple Grammy Award winner had become anorexic. The best explanation may be that of lyricist John Bettis, who told the *L.A. Times*, "My feeling is that everything came so naturally to Karen—the singing and even the dancing on a television special—that she felt she was *earning* her stardom by denying herself food."

Nicole Brown Simpson and Ronald Goldman

Near midnight on June 12, 1994, Nicole Brown Simpson, 35, and Ronald Goldman, 25, were found slashed to death outside the former's West Los Angeles condo. When the prime suspect in the slayings turned out to be former football star O. J. Simpson, and Judge Lance Ito allowed television cameras in court, the case riveted the nation.

At the trial, the coroner, Dr. Lakshmanan Sathyavagiswaran, determined it was likely the same knife was used to murder both victims and that both could have been slaughtered within minutes of each other. Further testimony provided hours of DNA analysis, familiarizing many viewers for the first time with this forensic science. DNA linked Simpson to the blood found at the Bundy Drive murder site.

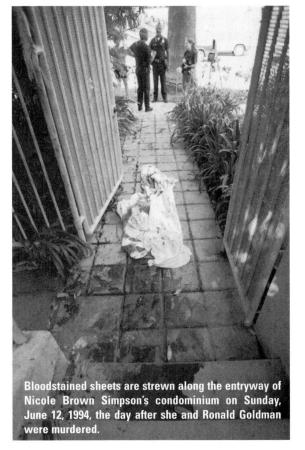

Bloodstained sheets are strewn along the entryway of Nicole Brown Simpson's condominium on Sunday, June 12, 1994, the day after she and Ronald Goldman were murdered.

Although the cause of death was clear, the time of death was not. While many legal analysts found enough forensic evidence to indict Simpson, there were disturbing discrepancies, which generated the defense's suggestion of an LAPD frame-up: The jailhouse nurse drew 8 cc's of Simpson's blood, but only 6.5 cc's could be accounted for. Detective Tom Vannater was carrying Simpson's blood sample at the murder scene, not having immediately booked it as evidence. EDTA, a preservative for blood samples, was found on a sock in Simpson's bedroom.

Simpson was found not guilty in criminal proceedings, but the legal action and public opinion that followed has ensnared him. Found guilty in the civil trial, Simpson was purportedly bankrupt.

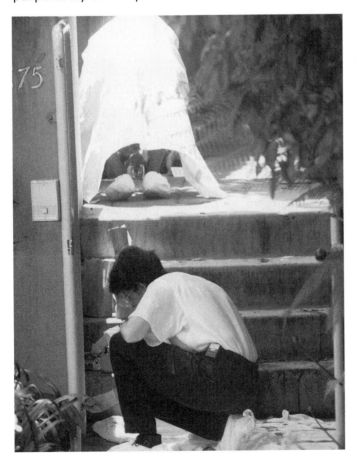

Ron Goldman's father, Fred, made unparalleled efforts in the media to plead for justice for his son. But what was actually known about the male victim in the case?

Ron Goldman liked to surf and give tennis lessons. Then he landed a string of waiting jobs that led to a position at Malibu's Pierview restaurant, where new friends ushered him into the Westside party scene. Although he still lived with his parents, and had no car and little money, he spent

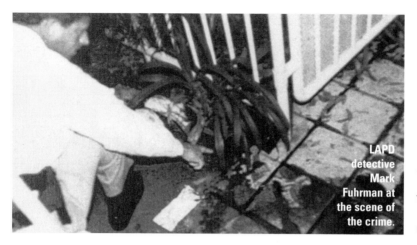

LAPD detective Mark Fuhrman at the scene of the crime.

spare afternoons playing beach volleyball and nights hitting L.A. hot spots, often paying no cover because he and his friends knew the bouncers. At one dance club in 1992, he met a leggy blonde who led Goldman deeper into the scene.

Their relationship grew serious enough for them to share an apartment in a Brentwood neighborhood populated with pockets of struggling actors, models, and musicians, while a few miles away, in the Hollywood Hills, loomed the mansions of the successful.

Goldman landed a waiting job at the California Pizza Kitchen in Brentwood which financed a day-to-day lifestyle of lifting weights at health clubs, quaffing lattes at Starbucks, socializing after work, and trying to figure out what to do with his life. When he and his girlfriend separated after a year, Goldman landed another table-waiting job at the casual but upscale Mezzaluna. He set out to learn the ways of the food-service industry and worked part-time as a promoter at local dance clubs, hoping the two gigs would lend him the experience to someday open his own joint.

During the day, he and his buddies maintained their ritual of pumping iron at The Gym, the same health club where O. J. Simpson paid $75 an hour to work out with a personal trainer. Goldman and his gang shelled out $50 a month to use the equipment. Afterward, they'd knock back java at Starbucks, sometimes chatting with Nicole Brown Simpson, O.J.'s ex-wife, who would drop in after her morning jog.

Although there was a 10-year gap in their ages, they hit it off, and soon Goldman could be seen cruising the streets in Nicole Brown Simpson's white Ferrari convertible and accompanying her to ritzy restaurants. When friends queried, Goldman insisted the relationship remained platonic. Whether it was or not, Goldman agreed that piloting the Ferrari with the beautiful, older blonde in the passenger seat gave him a giddy rush.

On the evening of June 12, Nicole and her two children and younger sister dined at Mezzaluna to celebrate her separation from Simpson. Goldman was working that night, but not serving their table. Around 10:00 P.M., Nicole phoned the restaurant to say she had left her glasses behind, and Goldman volunteered to take the misplaced spectacles to her condo, located only blocks away. Shortly after midnight, on June 13, they were found slashed to death on the walkway leading to her townhouse.

Within three days, the homicide squad gathered enough evidence to name Simpson a suspect. Key forensic findings included a bloody glove at O.J.'s Brentwood mansion that matched the one discovered at the murder scene; bloodstains in Simpson's white Ford Bronco, at his home, and at his ex-wife's condo; and a match between Simpson's blood type and blood at the murder site.

Told he would be arrested, Simpson asked to surrender at a specific time, then fled, embarking on the infamous, internationally televised, slow-speed freeway chase that concluded at his estate where he surrendered. The driver of Simpson's Bronco, former Buffalo Bills teammate A. C. Cowlings, was never questioned in court.

Seven months after Simpson pleaded not guilty and hired the most expensive legal defense team in history, the superhyped "trial of the century" began. A carnival-like atmosphere enveloped the downtown Criminal Courts Building, resembling a medieval execution scene, when mobs thronged the gallows to gawk at the condemned and hawk religious relics. This time, concessionaires peddled tacky trial T-shirts, cheap watches, souvenir books, and gaudy oil paintings of the infamous defendant, while perched on corners, evangelicals spouted admonitions of fire and brimstone.

By the trial's end, the *Los Angeles Times* had run over 1,500 articles on the case, 398 of them gracing the front page. *USA Today* featured 143 front-page Simpson stories. *Newsweek* magazine splashed his mug across the cover six times, while *Time* was admonished for purposely darkening a cover photo of Simpson for more dramatic impact. Certain reporters were so pressured to get new information from principal attorneys, they followed them into the men's rest rooms at the Criminal Courts Building.

In the end, a committee of the American Bar Association said media coverage of the Simpson trial "was the most spectacular and depressing example of improper publicity and professional misconduct ever presented to the people of the U.S. in a criminal trial."

Inaccuracies included reports of a second suspect arrested, a bloody ski mask at the murder scene, a blood-covered murder weapon in O.J.'s golf bag, and bloodstained clothes in O.J.'s washing machine.

Before the trial concluded, 35 books on the case had emerged from gleeful publishing houses, including best-sellers by Simpson (*I Want to Tell You*) and Faye Resnick, Nicole's close friend, whose gossipy account painted a bleak portrait of all involved. Two jurors evicted during the trial had tell-all books on newsstands, as did O.J.'s former houseguest, the would-be celebrity Brian Kato Kalin.

In the end, it seemed the only sympathetic witness in connection with the killings was Alan Park, who drove Simpson's limousine on the night of the crime. Park, who testified he saw a shadowy figure run into Simpson's mansion as Park waited outside, refused $60,000 from tabloid television show *A Current Affair* because "I didn't feel it was right to make substantial sums of money for yourself off two people's deaths."

Dr. Thomas Noguchi, "Coroner to the Stars"

The public knew him as the "coroner to the stars." He performed the autopsies on Marilyn Monroe, Robert Kennedy, and Sharon Tate, and supervised the investigations into the deaths of Janis Joplin, John Belushi, Natalie Wood, William Holden, and many other Hollywood glitterati. He invented a method to identify trace metals left by bullets in bodies that is now used throughout the nation. And he is the world's only medical examiner to have written a best-selling autobiography, *Coroner*, published in 1983. But most importantly, during his 15-year reign from 1967 to 1982 as chief medical examiner-coroner of Los Angeles County, the charismatic Dr. Thomas T. Noguchi turned the L.A. Coroner's Office into a world-class forensic science institution.

Born in 1927 in Tokyo, Japan, Noguchi was the oldest son of an aspiring artist who at the late age of 33 decided to become a doctor. A free-spirited boy and clever student, he got an unexpected lesson in the value of forensic medicine shortly after he turned 13. His father was charged with malpractice after a young man he was treating for strep throat died. The man's parents claimed their son had choked to death on a cotton swab Noguchi's father carelessly left in his patent's throat. To refute the charges, Noguchi's father asked that a court-appointed physician perform an autopsy, a very rare procedure in 1930s Japan. But the autopsy cleared him of the charges and left a lasting impression on his teenage son.

At 20, Noguchi enrolled at Tokyo's Nippon Medical School, and the next year entered law school concurrently, studying medicine by day and legal affairs at night. He graduated from medical school in 1951 and interned at Tokyo University Hospital, all the while

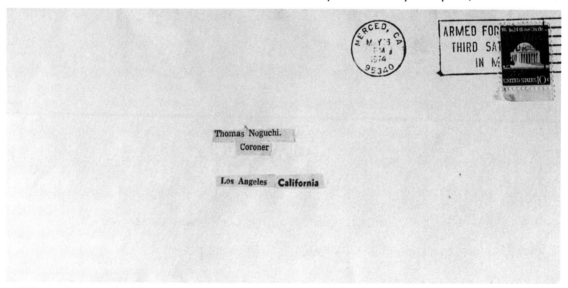

This envelope contained the **WANTED BY THE SLA** death threat sent to Dr. Noguchi by the Symbionese Liberation Army (see p. 141). Dr. Noguchi, whose staff protected him from crank letters, never saw the poster or envelope.

dreaming about learning firsthand the cutting-edge medicine practiced in America. The next year, he jumped at the chance to intern at the Orange County General Hospital, located just south of Los Angeles. In 1960, despite his peers' warnings that he was dooming himself to a low-paying career, Noguchi joined the L.A. Coroner's Office as a deputy medical examiner.

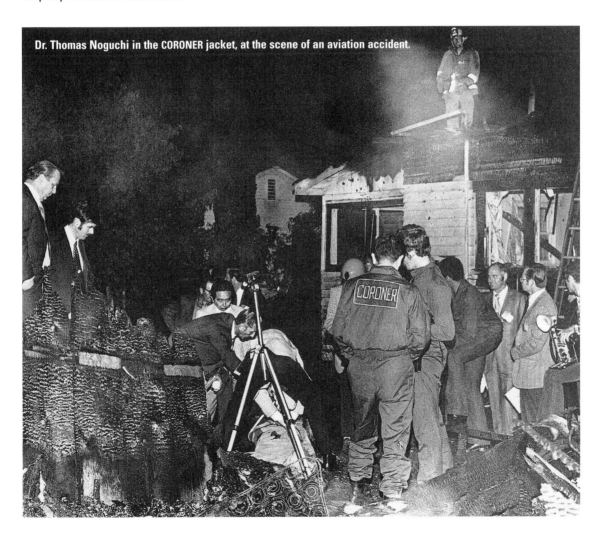

Dr. Thomas Noguchi in the CORONER jacket, at the scene of an aviation accident.

He quickly earned a reputation as a gifted and hard-driving pathologist, often working seven days straight, sometimes conducting autopsies until 3:00 A.M., before heading home to his new wife. In 1967, after a mere seven years with the department, he was named chief medical examiner-coroner.

As department head, Noguchi championed the building of a new coroner's facility that would contain the latest state-of-the-art technology and boost forensic medicine to the next plateau. The outdated, overcrowded, and ill-equipped coroner's quarters in the Hall of Justice basement represented the old style of determining cause of death. What Noguchi and his backers envisioned was not only creating a new facility but also a fresh approach to cause-of-death examinations. Called "total investigation," it would bring together under one roof investigators, criminalists, pathologists, and forensic scientists from various disciplines. The vision became reality on May 22, 1972, when the doors to the four-story Los Angeles County Forensic Science Center opened, a feat Noguchi saw as his crowning achievement.

Staffed with expert scientists and equipped with top instrumentation, the refitted Coroner's Office received requests from around the globe for help in unexplained deaths and mass disasters. For a two-year period in 1975–76, the L.A. Coroner took on an unprecedented 32 cases outside the county. In one instance, the Federal Aviation Administration flew the charred, unrecognizable remains of victims from a Pan American plane crash on the Pacific Island of Pago Pago to the Forensic Science Center to be identified.

For all his strengths, Noguchi was not beyond controversy. In 1969, after only two years at the helm, the Los Angeles County Board of Supervisors moved to discharge him for using his position as "an avenue of aggrandizement," among other charges. Backed by a groundswell of public support, Noguchi successfully rebutted the charges. In 1982, the year he was voted president of the National Association of Medical Examiners, the board moved to demote Noguchi, citing mismanagement among the charges. At the civil service hearing that followed, Noguchi's detractors criticized him as too visible and too much of a visionary to adequately supervise the department's day-to-day operations. Although he was demoted, Noguchi's legacy still remains intact.

CHAPTER 4

Spotlight on Forensics

They told me, Francis Hensley, they told me you were hung
With red protruding eye-balls and black protruding tongue.

I wept and I remembered how often you and I
had laughed about Los Angeles and now 'tis here you'll lie.

Here pickled in formaldehyde and painted like a whore,
Shrimp-pink, incorruptible, not lost or gone before.

—Evelyn Waugh, *The Loved One*

If Hollywood gave the L.A. County Department of Coroner global notoriety, forensic medicine and science has brought it worldwide fame. As medical detectives, forensic pathologists scrutinize corpses for clues indicating the manner, cause, and circumstances of death. They also examine anonymous bodies for signs, like a scar or a chipped tooth, that can lead to their identification.

Above all, forensic pathologists want to know if deaths stem from accidents or foul play. If foul play is involved, they can help bring justice by determining how, when, and

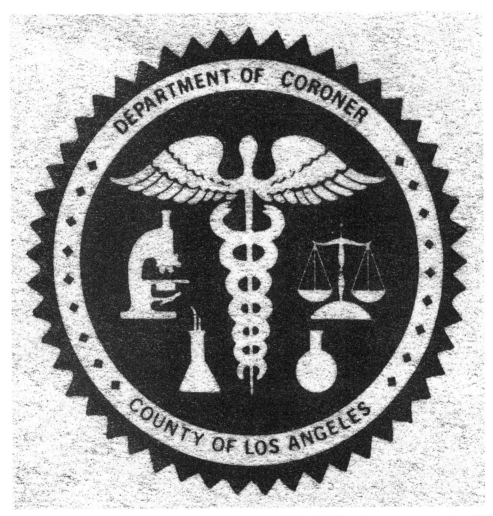

The design of the present-day logo was suggested by Dr. Noguchi in 1966. The microscope represents pathology; the beakers represent toxicology; the scales stand for law; and the winged staff symbolizes medical science.

where the death took place. Homicides typically reflect the killer's mind-set, and by knowing the method of homicide, police can create a psychological profile that may lead to a suspect.

For each coroner's case, a forensic pathologist leads the investigation into the cause of death, while various experts focus on their areas of specialty:

FORENSIC TOXICOLOGY: Forensic toxicologists analyze autopsy specimens, from blood to stomach contents, to determine if drugs, poisons, or other chemicals were involved in the cause or manner of death.

CRIMINALISTICS: Criminalists study trace evidence such as hair, bloodstains, fingernails, and fibers to help determine cause of death. They also use a scanning electron microscope to examine the gunshot residue left by cartridge primer particles on the hands, and the marks made on bones by murder tools such as knives. With these clues, they can characterize whether a suicide or homicide occurred.

HISTOPATHOLOGY: Pathologists scrutinize microscopic samples of tissue from muscles, skin, cartilage, nerves, and other organs for structural damage or disease that may have led to death.

NEUROPATHY:	Neuropathlogists examine and dissect brain and spinal cord tissue for damage to the nerve cell structure that may indicate cause of death.
FORENSIC ANTHROPOLOGY:	At scenes of mass disasters or burial sites of homicide victims, forensic anthropologists recover the skeletal remains. In the laboratory, they first analyze the bones to determine if the remains are of forensic interest or are ancient Indian remains. If the remains are of forensic interest, the forensic anthropologists determine the victim's age, race, and stature, and can provide clues to the cause of death.
ODONTOLOGY:	Forensic dentists compare the teeth of unknown corpses with dental records to determine their identities. They also study bite marks in both the flesh and the possessions of homicide victims to help identify the murderer.

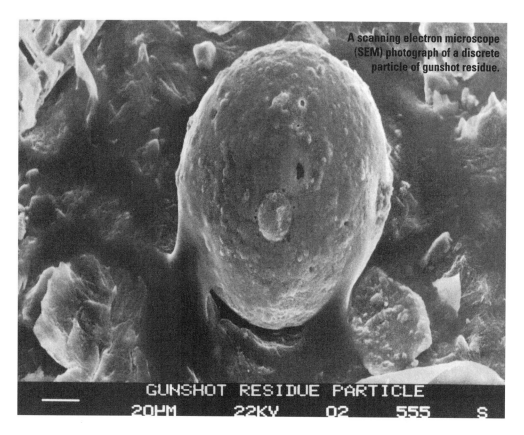

A scanning electron microscope (SEM) photograph of a discrete particle of gunshot residue.

GUNSHOT RESIDUE PARTICLE
20µM   22KV   02   555   S

Forensics in Action

Although the L.A. Coroner boasts a world-class forensics laboratory today, it wasn't always so. The coroner's rise to prominence, like that of Los Angeles, began after World War II. Back in the 1940s, when L.A. dallied as a sunbaked movie town, the Coroner's Office was crammed into the basement of the Hall of Justice, a poorly ventilated space where formaldehyde fumes swirled with the stench of decomposing bodies. By the 1960s, as L.A.'s population surged, the coroner clamored for a larger, upgraded facility. These needs were met in 1972 when the Coroner's Office moved into the glistening, new Los Angeles County Forensics Science Center, which quickly became a hotbed of forensic development.

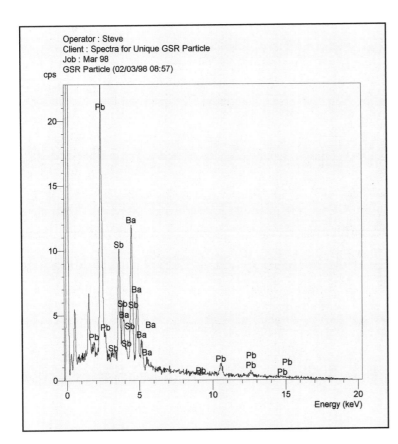

Operator : Steve
Client : Spectra for Unique GSR Particle
Job : Mar 98
GSR Particle (02/03/98 08:57)

This spectra for the SEM photograph on page 166 shows the chemical composition of the discrete particle to be prime material from a bullet cartridge. Such particles, if found on the hands of a victim, can indicate suicide; if found on a suspect's hands, they can be supporting evidence of guilt in a homicide.

With its team of experts, the L.A. Coroner has become a role model for disaster responses as well as a pivotal player in solving some of the county's most infamous crimes. Bullet-riddled bodies, midair collisions, serial slayings—it's the coroner's mission to straighten out the region's wreckage. The following cases illustrate the way different specialists from the coroner's team of forensic scientists and investigators unlock the mysteries surrounding the cause of death.

Odontology Case No. 1:
The Night Stalker

On October 4, 1989, Richard Ramirez, the so-called "Night Stalker," was sentenced to death for 13 murders, 11 sexual assaults, and 14 burglaries. This climaxed one of the largest police investigations and longest criminal trials in Los Angles history at the time. In both, forensic dentistry played a significant role.

The Night Stalker crimes occurred between June 1984 and August 1985, all linked by "signature clues" such as entry through sliding doors, the cutting of phone cords, the drawing of pentagrams (satanic symbols), and footprints of Avia tennis shoes. Another common thread was the extraordinary brutality. In one instance, a woman was raped on the floor near her dead husband, then bound and forced to remain nearby as the attacker sodomized her 8-year-old son.

With one exception, surviving witnesses said their attacker had stained and gapped teeth. A police artist, using witness descriptions, created a dental illustration that was included in the Night Stalker police bulletin.

On June 15, 1985, the Night Stalker narrowly escaped capture. The police stopped a car for running a stop sign, but the driver leapt from the vehicle and outran the officers. In the car, police found a business card of a Los Angeles dentist, who later told investigators he had treated a patient named Richard Mena who fit the vague description of the

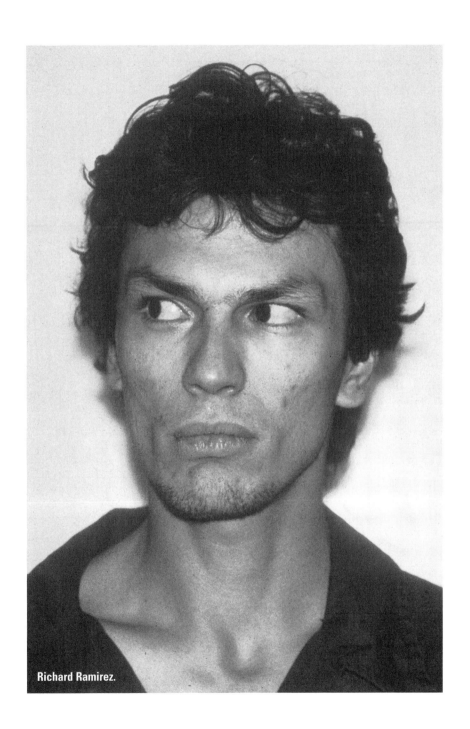

Richard Ramirez.

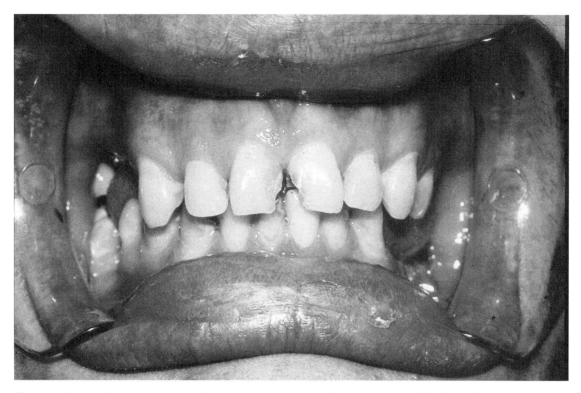

fleeing driver. More importantly, the dentist's detailed portrait of Richard Mena matched witness descriptions of the Night Stalker. The dentist handed over Mena's dental charts and X rays, and that August, a police investigator gave them to the coroner's chief forensic dentist, Dr. Gerald Vale, who created a dental description for the police bulletin.

About two weeks later, the police, using fingerprints, identified the Night Stalker as a drifter from Texas named Richard Ramirez and released a photo of him to the news media. Less than 12 hours later, on the morning of August 31, he was seized by an enraged crowd in the Latino community of Boyle Heights after he had attacked a young woman and tried to steal her car.

Shortly after Ramirez was jailed, Dr. Vale, accompanied by Dr. Betty Hoffman, examined his teeth in the prison dental offices. During the inquiry, Ramirez was amiable and talkative, explaining that his condition of decaying and missing teeth stemmed from a steady diet of junk food and sodas. Near the session's end, as Dr. Vale was taking photographs, he saw Ramirez become suddenly hostile, clenching and unclenching his fists and scraping the floor with his foot. Realizing the hotheaded man on the other side of the camera was charged with 13 murders, the dentist quickly called the attending deputy sheriff, who took Ramirez into the hall and stood by as he vented his rage by furiously kicking the wall.

Later, Dr. Vale compared the dental information from his examination of Ramirez to the dental records of Richard Mena and found they were exactly the same.

At Ramirez's trial, the defense raised the question of mistaken identity. On the witness stand, Ramirez's father claimed his son was in Texas when three of the Night Stalker crimes were committed. The prosecution countered by calling the Los Angeles dentist who had treated Richard Mena. The dentist testified he had examined Mena during the time period that the father claimed his son to be in Texas, and he stated he recognized Ramirez as the man who called himself "Richard Mena." Next, the prosecution called the coroner's chief forensic dentist, Dr. Vale, who testified that dental records show Richard Ramirez and Richard Mena were, beyond any doubt, the same man.

Odontology Case No. 2: Midair Collision

On August 30, 1986, at 11:55 A.M., in the skies above the affluent L.A. suburb of Cerritos, a single-engine Piper clipped the tail of an Aeromexico DC-9, sending both planes careening out of control and crashing in a massive fireball that hurled flaming wreckage across tiled roofs, manicured lawns, and luxury cars. All passengers and personnel on both planes perished, while flying debris killed more than a dozen residents and visitors in Cerritos. The death toll was 83.

Within the hour, the coroner's disaster response team began scouring the crash site for dismembered bodies, which they sent to the Forensics Science Center for identification. The Piper's pilot was among the first found, his body intact and in condition for an autopsy. By examining samples of his heart tissue under a microscope, pathologists determined the pilot had probably suffered a nonfatal cardiac arrest moments before hitting the DC-9. With this knowledge, aviation authorities speculated that the pilot may have been unconscious or too weak to maneuver his plane out of the jetliner's flight path.

Meanwhile, as charred remains poured into the Forensics Science Center, odontologists x-rayed the crash victims' teeth, while the coroner's staff tried to obtain the passengers' dental records. Once the records were received, odontologists compared them to the postmortem X rays to identify the victims. Unfortunately, this proved difficult because many of the Mexicans aboard had no dental records. In those cases, forensic anthropologists could only determine the victim's race, sex, and stature. Nonetheless, the coroner's staff identified over 80 percent of the remains within weeks.

Odontology Case No. 3: Airport Disaster

On the evening of February 1, 1991, a USAir Boeing 737 approached Los Angeles International Airport (LAX) and was mistakenly cleared to land. As it touched down, the jet struck a Skywest Metroliner commuter plane that had been instructed to taxi onto the same runway on which the larger plane was landing. The 737 dragged the commuter craft over a quarter mile before crashing into an abandoned fire station and bursting into flames.

The Metroliner was so completely demolished that rescue workers were unaware a second plane was involved until they had extinguished the fire and noticed a propeller under the wreckage of the 737.

Somehow, 67 people aboard the 737 escaped the blaze, while 22 perished. All 12 aboard the Metroliner died. It was the worst disaster in the bustling international airport's history.

The coroner's disaster response team soon arrived to remove the bodies and identify each victim. However, the operation was delayed two days until emergency workers could dislodge the 4,000 gallons of aviation fuel threatening to ignite.

On February 3, the coroner's crew began easing bodies from the wreckage. As each victim was extricated, a forensic dentist examined the mouth to ensure the teeth and jaw were intact so the body could be identified. Meanwhile, a forensic anthropologist, Dr. Judy Suchey, raked the wreckage for minute pieces of human remains.

For most victims, fire and trauma had destroyed fingerprints and recognizable features, making teeth and jaw structure the only way to identify them. While the recovery operation continued, the coroner's staff worked with the airlines to obtain the dental records of all believed to have been aboard both planes. Forensic dentists then matched the records to the victims' dental structures, comparing characteristics such as tooth position, root shape, crown shape, dental work, and missing teeth. By February 7, all the victims had been identified, with 22 of the 34 distinguished by dental evidence.

Investigative Case No. I: Patio Tomb

In the early 1990s, a new homeowner was removing an old cement patio in his backyard when he discovered a body encased in the slab of concrete. The cement with the body inside was taken to the Coroner's Forensic Science Center where the casting was carefully removed from the remains.

It turned out that whoever poured the cement had mixed it at very watery consistency, and as it dried over the body, it created an impression of a woman's face and hands that was detailed enough to identify the victim. Using the impressions left in the cement, a coroner's investigator discovered the previous homeowner was also the decedent's husband. He became the prime suspect.

Investigative Case No. 2: A Foul Trunk

In 1994, a storage company auctioned off three trunks, after their owner failed to pay his long-overdue balance. When the high bidder went to collect the chests, he smelled foul odors emanating from them and called the police. In each of the trunks, the police discovered a decaying body.

Shortly after, the trunks' original owner, unaware his belongings had been sold, asked the storage company if he could resume making storage payments. The company encouraged him to do so and called the homicide detectives. They arrested him when he came to make the back payments.

Toxicology Case No. 1: A Quiet Killer

In the early 1980s, a new street drug mimicking the effects of morphine and similar narcotics was detected in overdose victims in counties surrounding Los Angeles, although there were no cases in L.A. County. The drug, alpha-methylfentany, combined with other closely related compounds, was so overwhelmingly potent that an overdose could occur in the minuscule picogram range (a billionth of a gram per milliliter of blood). Drug users, however, treated it as if it were a just another type of heroin.

Medical examiners from outlying counties were baffled by deaths that had the symptoms of a narcotics overdose but revealed nothing in the toxicology tests. When the forensic toxicologists found no trace of drugs, they suspected alpha-methylfentany to be the culprit and sent blood and tissue samples to the University of California, Davis, toxicology laboratory, whose highly sophisticated equipment could in fact detect minuscule levels of this elusive substance.

Criminalistics Case No. 1: A Telltale Cocktail

In the summer of 1986, a coroner's senior criminalist examined the stomach contents of a 25-year-old woman who had been strangled to death. The criminalist discovered the remains of mushrooms, water chestnuts, pickles, pepper seeds, and pineapples. When she told the detectives investigating the case of her findings, they reasoned that the unusual fruit and vegetable mixture may have been the ingredients of an exotic, tropical drink. Following this lead, the detectives investigated bars in the area where the strangulation victim was found to see if any served cocktails with the telltale ingredients.

Eventually, they came across a nightspot that made a tropical concoction called a "Suffering Bastard," a mixed drink containing pineapple juice, honey, sweet and sour sauce, orange juice, pickle garnish, and rum, consistent with the victim's stomach contents. They'd found their bar.

After interviewing the bartender and patrons there on the night of the murder, the detectives were able to identify and apprehend the suspect.

Criminalistics Case No. 2: Seed of Knowledge

In the early 1980s, a young woman of Middle Eastern origin was found dead in a cloth suitcase at Los Angeles International Airport (LAX). With no identification on the body, the only information investigators could locate was that the suitcase had been in the cargo hold of a direct flight to LAX from Frankfurt, Germany.

Shortly after that body had been discovered, the body of young man of Middle Eastern descent was found in a car in San Francisco with a gunshot wound to the head in an apparent suicide.

Back in Los Angeles, a coroner's senior criminalist examined the suitcase and discovered a watermelon seed that was traced to a specific strain grown only in the area of Tehran, Iran. In San Francisco, investigators found identification on the man's person and documents showing he'd been aboard a flight from Tehran to Frankfurt. After contacting Iranian officials, investigators determined that the female decedent and the male decedent were husband and wife.

Apparently, the couple had been determined to get to America, but since only the husband had a passport, he smuggled his wife into the country by stowing her in the suitcase. When he learned she had died—from positional asphyxia or suffocation—he committed suicide.

EPILOGUE

The Coroner in the Community

While it's the coroner's legal duty to determine cause of death, the Los Angeles County Department of Coroner has stepped up its operations to extend far beyond this mandate. Over the years, it has set up numerous programs to serve the county, corralling its resources to counsel wayward teens, train medical students in forensic pathology, and supply certain tissues to low-income hospital patients. Today, the L.A. Coroner runs more than 16 community service programs, a number that will rise to meet tomorrow's needs.

Disaster Preparation and Response makes the Coroner among the first county agencies to respond to multideath emergencies such as airplane crashes and earthquakes. First, the department helps plan how the county will react to catastrophes; and in the field, it oversees the recovery, storage, and identification of the victims.

The Youthful Drunk Driver Visitation Program plays a pivotal role in the county's efforts to reform first offenders on probation for driving under the influence of alcohol or drugs. Implemented by the Coroner's Office in 1989, the program involves working with municipal courts, area hospitals, and alcohol treatment facilities to deter persons convicted of driving under the influence from becoming repeat offenders. Since then, the program has been expanded to include other offenses, such as weapons-related offenses, domestic violence, drug-related offenses, and other vehicle code violations. The crux of the program revolves around showing young offenders firsthand the devastation caused by their behavior to their victims and the victims' families. This is done by giving them a tour of their local hospital and the Coroner's facility.

At the Coroner's Office, the participants learn about and discuss the effects of alcohol

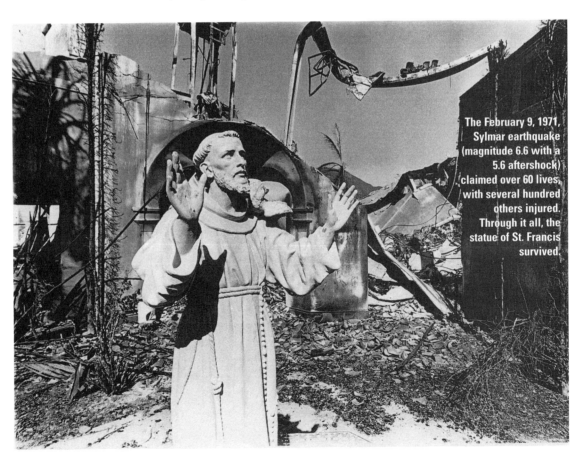

The February 9, 1971, Sylmar earthquake (magnitude 6.6 with a 5.6 aftershock) claimed over 60 lives, with several hundred others injured. Through it all, the statue of St. Francis survived.

and drugs on their lives and others, including possible consequences such as child endangerment, suicide, and murder. Next, they are shown a slide presentation graphically illustrating the all-too-common results of driving under the influence and other effects of violence. Finally, they are given a tour of the coroner's facility that includes the service floor, where participants are shown dead bodies of people who were the victims of these crimes. Over the course of its eight-year history, the program has proved a successful deterrent.

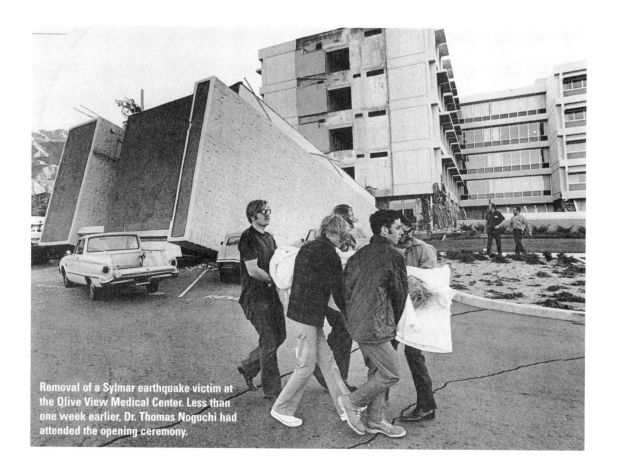

Removal of a Sylmar earthquake victim at the Olive View Medical Center. Less than one week earlier, Dr. Thomas Noguchi had attended the opening ceremony.

Tissue Harvesting and Organ Transplantation enables the coroner, with the consent of the decedents' families, to provide selected tissues, such as corneas, skin, and bone, to federally chartered tissue banks and make them available to low-income patients at county hospitals free of charge.

The Los Angeles County Interagency Scuba Committee allows the coroner to work with other county agencies to investigate scuba diving fatalities and develop ways to help prevent future scuba diving accidents. Underwater deaths contribute significantly to the number of sporting fatalities in this region, well known for its population of outdoor enthusiasts.

The Interagency Council on Child Abuse and Neglect (ICAN) is an

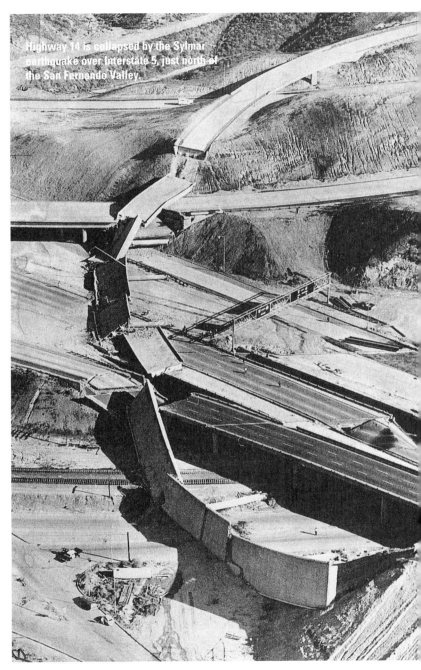

Highway 14 is collapsed by the Sylmar earthquake over Interstate 5, just north of the San Fernando Valley.

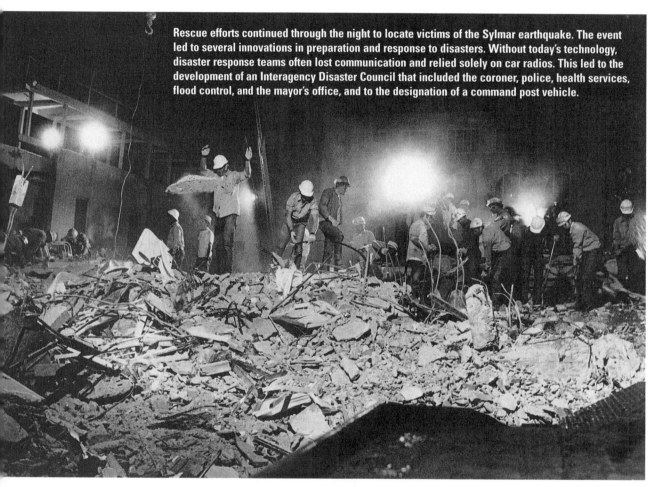

Rescue efforts continued through the night to locate victims of the Sylmar earthquake. The event led to several innovations in preparation and response to disasters. Without today's technology, disaster response teams often lost communication and relied solely on car radios. This led to the development of an Interagency Disaster Council that included the coroner, police, health services, flood control, and the mayor's office, and to the designation of a command post vehicle.

agency in which the coroner plays an active role. Members of the coroner's staff sit on the ICAN committee that investigates the questionable deaths of children.

The SIDS Program allows the coroner to participate in the Interagency Council on Sudden Infant Death Syndrome. The coroner's staff has developed standards for investigating SIDS deaths and conducting autopsies. The state has made SIDS-related data collection a top priority.

The Visiting Physician Scholar Program hosts renowned physicians from throughout the world at the Forensic Science Center. Staying up to two years, the physicians learn the latest in forensic methods and the recent developments in conducting autopsies. The guest physicians also perform autopsies under staff supervision.

The Residency Program offers graduate medical students training in forensic pathology and prepares aspiring deputy medical examiners for board certification. Under close supervision, participants perform the various functions in cause-of-death determinations. This program is approved by the Accreditation Council for Graduate Education.

University Hospitals Pathology Resident Training Program lets pathology residents from local university-affiliated hospitals, such as L.A. County–USC Medical Center and the UCLA Medical Center, work side by side with experienced forensic scientists in cause-of-death determinations.

Nursing Home Deaths is a state-mandated program that decrees the coroner examine all reportable deaths occurring in certain convalescent facilities.

Identification of Unidentified Bodies is another state-mandated program in which the coroner participates in a California-wide effort to identify all John and Jane Does, regardless of where they met their demise.

Contract Programs involves the coroner in a variety of legal and medical operations. The coroner conducts drug tests for the probation department, HIV testing for the county, and blood–alcohol analysis for the courts. It also participates in a host of state- and federally subsidized studies. Most recently, the coroner has worked with state agencies to analyze the spread of HIV cases and with the Commerce Department to examine the link between highway accidents and the abuse of methamphetamines by long-distance truck drivers.

MECAP–Medical Board of California Reporting Function are statewide consumer safety programs. The Coroner's Office keeps a tally of county deaths stemming from unsafe consumer products and those directly related to negligent doctors. The Office then presents its findings to Sacramento.

With its ever-expanding list of community service programs, the Coroner's Office seeks to lower the number of sudden and violent deaths that comprise its caseload. And this pursuit has made the coroner more than an investigator into the cause of death: It is also a guardian of life.

Ultimately, it is the Department of Coroner's role to give life a sense of closure, guaranteeing that the deceased has an identity, a grave site, and a proper burial. It uses the best of modern science to perform this task that is as ancient and sacred as the human race. Wherever they fall and however they die in this jumbled desert city that sprawls along the sea, the L.A. Coroner will continue to pick up the pieces and put them to rest. More than any other discipline, the Coroner remains the advocate for the deceased.

Skeletons in the Closet

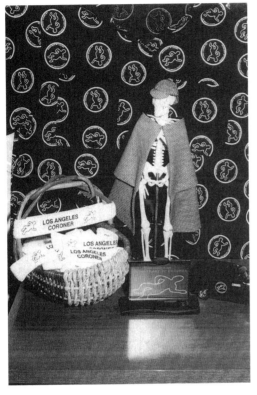

He's thin, lanky, puffs a pipe, and proudly sports a deerstalker cap. And he has no flesh.

Meet Sherlock, the official mascot of Skeletons in the Closet, the Los Angeles County Coroner's gift shop and mail-order merchandising program. As you flip through the world's first and only Coroner memorabilia catalogue, you'll find toe tag key chains, a coin bank shaped like the "Black Mariah" (a 1930s coroner's van), coffee mugs stamped with the grinning image of Sherlock, "undertakers" (boxer shorts decorated with body outlines like those drawn by police around homicide victims), and the ever-popular beach towels bearing a body outline.

Located at the Forensics Science Center, Skeletons in the Closet opened in September 1993. Proceeds go to underwrite the aforementioned community and outreach programs, including the Visiting Physician Scholar Program, which otherwise would have been cut for lack of funding. The business quickly surpassed expectations, with

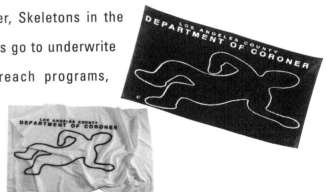

gross sales exceeding $100,000 in its first year and currently approaching $750,000 annually. The number of items offered has soared from 6 to over 50 today.

Interest in products from the coroner that handles Hollywood's infamous deaths has proven particularly popular overseas. Skeletons in the Closet has been featured by magazines and newspapers in England, France, Germany, Australia, Hong Kong, and South Africa. Recently, a Japanese firm paid $30,000 for the rights to license and distribute merchandise with the L.A. Coroner's logo in Japan. Every day, tourists stop by to examine the goods, many saying they're on their way to Disneyland. Angelenos drop in as well. After completing *Interview With the Vampire*, Brad Pitt spent part of an afternoon browsing among the undertakers and toe tags while researching his role for the movie *Seven*.

For their part, the coroner's staff prefer to sell items that mix amusement and caution, such as the toe tag key chains, which offer a bit of gallows humor with a warning against driving under the influence. (A free mail-order catalogue may be obtained by calling 213/343-0760 or writing to Skeletons in the Closet, 1104 North Mission Road, Los Angeles, CA 90033.)

Skeletons in the Closet symbolizes the irony of the Coroner's Office. It would seem to be a place for the grimmest and most unrewarding of tasks. Yet, in researching files there, we found it is a life-affirming place, whose employees exhibit a certain energy and sense of humor to countermand the surroundings.

Hollywood *Noir* and the Coroner

Since its inception, Los Angeles has been driven by a lust for cash and the good life it brings. The 1880s population boom quadrupled the number of the desert hamlet's inhabitants and laid the foundation for urbanization. The railroads, trying to spur ticket sales, commissioned the publisher of the *Los Angeles Star* to write travel articles promoting the small seaside town as a sunny paradise with a romantic Spanish past and glittering American future. The evocation of a sun-kissed utopia with orange trees and vineyards lured hundreds of thousands from the chills of the Midwest and Northeast. The railroads made a killing, while real estate moguls grew plump selling suburban plots to newcomers dreaming about creating new lives behind white picket fences.

No other city has had its downside so allegorized before the film camera as Los Angeles, from *The Big Sleep* to *L.A. Confidential*, with stops along the way for *The Loved One*, *True Confessions*, *Chinatown*, and *Pulp Fiction*, among others.

The coroner is a role player in this imagery, just as in real life. In *Chinatown*, the masterpiece of noir allegory on film, the theme of evil is not compromised. It is sustained throughout, right through to the final, bitter lines, heard over the wail of an automobile horn and the cries of a distraught, young woman, as her mother lies dead, slumped over the steering wheel with a bullet in her skull:

"Go home, Jake. It's Chinatown."

That final sense of the inevitability of death is part of the process for those who work in the Los Angeles County Department of Coroner. They deal with the deaths of not just the celebrated and infamous, but of all the Jane and John Does who have receded into the mists of time, whether by accident, by their own hands, or by the actions of others.

What seizes one, looking through the often grim, visceral photos and files in the Coroner's Office, is this: This is work that requires a passionate underpinning of humanity. The employees of the Coroner's Office are no less human and vulnerable than the rest of us. However, they use professionalism, a sense of social purpose, and, most of all, their reinforced sense of compassion to persevere.

There are those who cannot persevere, or those whose end is sudden, untimely. Perhaps, in the final analysis, it is the heightened expectations connected with L.A.'s lifestyle and opportunities, mixed with the irrevocable disappointments of life, that keep the Coroner's Office as busy as it is.

In Hans Holbein's 1538 *Dance of Death* woodcut series, the most scenic and gentle visitation by Death is reserved for the Ploughman.

As the aged and bent figure furrows his field, Death grasps the traces of his horses and eases the Ploughman's final journey, leading him sweetly toward a glorious sunset.

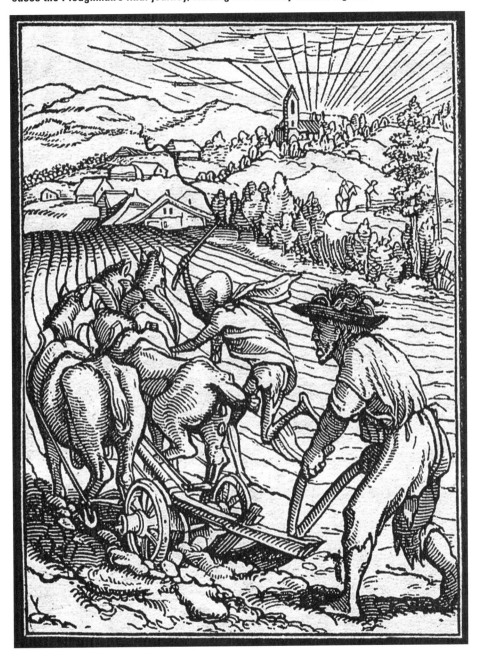

INDEX

P

Paramount Pictures, 82, 85-86
Pare, Ambroise, 27-28
Parent, Steven Earl, 130-31
Park, Alan, 157
Parker, Marion, 69-73, *71*
Parker, Perry, 69
pathology. *See* forensic science
Peters, Ernest, 92
Phoenix Program, The, 142
photography, 17
physician training, 41, 183
Pickford, Mary, 82
Pitt, Brad, 186
Pittluck, Norman, 136
Pitts, Zasu, 81
Polanski, Roman, 127
police corruption, 102, 104-5
Pollack, William Jerome, *109*
press coverage of deaths
    Herald Examiner, 98, 99, 101
    Illustrated Daily News, 81
    L.A. Mirror, 105
    Los Angeles Star, 50, 56
    Los Angeles Times, 156
    New York Herald, 56
    Newsweek, 156
    Rolling Stone, 135
    San Francisco Bulletin, 56
    USA Today, 156
Prinze, Freddie, 145-47
Private Diary of My Life With Lana, The, 111
Purkinje, Johannes, 28
Purviance, Edna, 83-84

Q

Questiones Medico Regales, 28
Quincy, 19, 20-21, 43-45

R

Ramirez, Richard, 168-171, *169*
Reagan, Ronald, President, 45, 141
Reeves, George, 113-15
Residency Programs, 183
Resnick, Faye, 157
Restrepo, Guillermo, 135
Richard the Lion-Hearted, 26-27
Rokitansky, Carl, 30
Root, Eric, 111
Rowland, W.R., Sheriff, 54
Rummel, Sam, *104*, 104-6

S

Salazar, Rubin, 134-37
Saltzer, Robert, 117
San Francisco Bulletin, 56
Sathyavagiswaran, Lakshmanan, M.D., 152
Schaefer, Walter, 117
scuba diving deaths, 181
Seale, Bobby, 144
Sebring, Jay, 128-29
Selig, William, 62
Shafer, Rudolf, *93*
Shelby, Charlotte, 87-88
Short, Elizabeth, *98*, 98-102, *100*
SIDS (Sudden Infant Death Syndrome)
    Program, 182
Siegel, Benjamin "Bugsy," *95-97*
Simpson, Nicole Brown, 152-57
Simpson, O. J., 152-57
Sirhan, Sirhan Bishara, 123, 124, *125*
Skeletons in the Closet, 185-86
SLA (Symbionese Liberation Army), 140-
    44, 158
Slatzer, Robert, 117, 118
Snyder, Marvin "Dusty," 145, 147
Sonney, Dan, 65
St. Francis Dam Disaster, 74-77, *75*
St. John, Adela Rogers, 88
stomach content analysis, 174-75
Stompanato, Johnny, 17, *107*, 107-13
Sturner, William, M.D., 121
Suchey, Judy, D.D.S., 172
suicide vs. accidental death
    Joplin, Janis, 137-39
    Prinze, Freddie, 145-47
suicides
    autopsy protocol, 18
    Great Depression-related, 37
    Medieval English law, 27
    Monroe, Marilyn, 115-19
    psychological autopsy, 32
suitcase, suffocation in, 175-76
Symbionese Liberation Army (SLA), 140-
    44, 158

T

Tabachnick, Norman, 116
Tate, Sharon, *127*, 127-31, 157
Taylor, William Desmond, 82-88
Thompson, Hunter S., 135
Thompson, Robert, 55
Todd, Thelma, 90-95, *91*, *92*
toxicology, 18, 28, *38*, 164, 175

transplantation, tissue/organ, 181
trunks storing corpses, 174-75
Tuck, Wong, M.D., 56
Turner, Lana, 17, 107-13, *108*

U

unidentified bodies, 41, 160, 170-72, 175-
    76, 183
Universal Studios, 63
University of California, Los Angeles, 53
USA Today, 156

V

Vale, Gerald, D.D.S., 170-71
Valentino, Douglas, 143
Van de Kamp, John, D.A., 118
Van Houten, Leslie, 131, 134
Van Ronkel, Carol, 113, 114
Vannater, Tom, 153
Vasquez, Tiburcio, *53*, 54
Virchow, Rudolf, 31
Visiting Physician Scholar Program, 183
voodoo ritual case, 41

W

Wagner, A. P., M.D., 90
Wallis, Bert, *92*
Ward, Lynn, 136
*Washing Away of Unjust Imputations or
    Wrongs, The*, 26
Watts riot, 12, 15
West, Roland, 90, 92, *93*, *94*
Whitehead, May, 90
Willis, Margaret, 67-68
Wilson, Thomas, 135, 137
woodcuts by Hans Holbein the Younger,
    22-23, 189
Woolwine, Thomas Lee, 87, 88

Y

Yakima Jim, 63
Younger, Evelle, D.A., 137
Yung, Sam, 55

Z

Zacchias, Paulo, 28
Zeehandelaar, Felix, 60
Zukor, Adolph, 84